Vedashree Sakhare
Savitha P.N

REHABILITATION OF MAXILLOFACIAL PROSTHESES MADE EASY WITH IMPLANTS

Vedashree Sakhare
Savitha P.N

REHABILITATION OF MAXILLOFACIAL PROSTHESES MADE EASY WITH IMPLANTS

LAP LAMBERT Academic Publishing

Imprint

Cover image: www.ingimage.com

Publisher:
LAP LAMBERT Academic Publishing
is a trademark of
Dodo Books Indian Ocean Ltd. and OmniScriptum S.R.L publishing group

120 High Road, East Finchley, London, N2 9ED, United Kingdom
Str. Armeneasca 28/1, office 1, Chisinau MD-2012, Republic of Moldova, Europe
Managing Directors: Ieva Konstantinova, Victoria Ursu
info@omniscriptum.com

Printed at: see last page
ISBN: 978-620-8-43981-1

Maxillofacial prostheses play a vital role in comprehensive rehabilitation by restoring physical and psychological well-being in patients with missing or disfigured anatomical structures due to congenital abnormalities, trauma, or disease .

Maxillofacial prosthetics defined by the current **Glossary of Prosthodontic Terms – GPT 10"** as the branch of Prosthodontics concerned with the restoration and/or replacement of the stomatognathic (jaws) and craniofacial (facial) structures with prostheses that may or may not be removed on a regular or elective basis".[1]

It is possible to restore esthetics, function and re-establish the self confidence of the patient by providing a well designed prosthesis such as a prosthetic ear, eye, nose, cranial plate or a combination of these. The last few decades have witnessed a significant increase in extensive malignancies of the head and neck region .

This has resulted in increasing number of patients with extensive post-surgical defects. Many of them need to be suitably rehabilitated to minimize long-term physical, functional and psychological consequences and ensure early return to normal life.

In addition, these patients could be more willing to accept large surgical resections, if counseled about prosthetic reconstruction, prior to definitive surgery. It is crucial that all such patients receive a pre-operative referral to a maxillofacial prosthodontist prior to surgery .

When these patients report to the maxillofacial prosthetic clinic they report with complex defects and their general health status is also compromised.

Achieving adequate retention of the prosthesis, especially when the defect is extensive, is a big challenge and requires a multi-disciplinary approach.

With the advent of predictable osseointegration, a new era dawned in the field of prosthodontic rehabilitation of the head and neck region.

Cases that were earlier condemned as “hopeless” were suddenly given a new range of options and the chance to be comprehensively restored to form and function.[2]

The aim of this library dissertation is to study about the different maxillofacial defects ,retention aids and role of implants used for the rehabilitation of the defects in detail.

The data regarding this topic was obtained from GOOGLE SCHOLAR, Pub Med , Scribd , International Journal Of Applied Dental Sciences, Hindawi ,Research Gate, Intech Open ,Science Direct , IP Annals Of Prosthodontics and Restorative Dentistry.

Out of 61 articles obtained ,47 articles are selected for my library dissertation.

- **Auricular prosthesis** : A removable maxillofacial prosthesis that artificially restores part of or the entire natural ear.
- **Biomaterial** : Substance that has been engineered to take a form which, alone or as part of a complex system, is used to direct, by control of interactions with components of living systems, the course of any therapeutic or diagnostic procedure, in human or veterinary medicine.
- **Craniofacial implants** : Implants that are used in the head and neck when traditional dental implants cannot be used due to minimal bone and risk to surrounding structures; a common location would be the temporal bone to support or retain an auricular prostheses.
- **Facial prosthesis**: A maxillofacial prosthesis that artificially replaces a deficient anatomy of the face as a result of surgery, trauma, or congenital absence.
- **Implant** : Any object or material, such as an alloplastic substance or other tissue, which is partially or completely inserted or grafted into the body for therapeutic, diagnostic, prosthetic, or experimental purposes.
- **Implant-supported prosthesis** : Dental prosthesis, such as artificial crown, fixed complete denture, fixed partial denture, removable complete overdenture, removable partial overdenture, as well as maxillofacial prosthesis, which are supported and retained in part or whole by dental implants.
- **Maxillofacial prosthesis** : Any prosthesis used to replace part or all of any stomatognathic and/or craniofacial structures.
- **Maxillofacial prosthetics** : The branch of prosthodontics concerned with the restoration and/or replacement of stomatognathic and craniofacial structures with prostheses that may or may not be removed on a regular or elective basis.
- **Nasal prosthesis** : A removable maxillofacial prosthesis that artificially restores the nose, partially or in its entirety.
- **Ocular prosthesis** : A maxillofacial prosthesis that artificially replaces an eye missing as a result of trauma, surgery, or congenital absence; the prosthesis does not replace missing eyelids or adjacent skin, mucosa or muscle.

- **Orbital prosthesis** : A maxillofacial prosthesis that artificially restores the eye, eyelids, and adjacent hard and soft tissues.
- **Osseointegration** : 1. The apparent direct attachment or connection of osseous tissue to an inert, alloplastic material without intervening fibrous connective tissue; 2. The process and resultant apparent direct connection of an exogenous material's surface and the host bone tissues, without intervening fibrous connective tissue present; 3. The interface between alloplastic materials and bone.
- **Polyvinyl siloxane** : An addition reaction silicone elastomeric impression material of silicone polymers having terminal vinyl groups that cross-link with silanes on activation by a platinum or palladium salt catalyst.
- **Retention** : That quality inherent in the dental prosthesis acting to resist the forces of dislodgment along the path of placement.[1]

HISTORY OF IMPLANTS USED IN MAXILLOFACIAL PROSTHESIS

The history of the evolution of dental implants is a rich and fascinating travelogue through time. Since the beginning of mankind, humans have used dental implants in one form or another to replace missing teeth.

In approximately 2500 BC, the ancient Egyptians tried to stabilize teeth that were periodontally involved with the use of ligature wire made of gold.

Artificial eyes, ears ,nose were found on Egyptian mummies.

AMBROSE PARE in 1517-1590 attempted to make ears made of paper and leather and method of securing them was by means of a head clip.

In 1728, PIERRE FAUCHARD designed a prostheses supported with wings that were positioned by patient from the oral side of obturator and made use of floor of nose for retention.[3]

In 1889, CLAUDE MARTIN , a French man illustrated a variety of prosthetic replacements including a particularly interesting attempt to retain a porcelain nose prosthesis with an intra oral mechanism.

In the 1700's, Dr. Hunter suggested transplanting teeth from one human to another; his experiment involved the implantation of an incompletely developed tooth into the comb of a rooster. He observed an extraordinary and astonishing event: the tooth became firmly embedded in the comb of the rooster and the blood vessels of the rooster grew straight into the pulp of the tooth.

In 1809, J. Maggiolo inserted a gold implant tube into a fresh extraction site.

This site was allowed to heal and then a crown was later added; unfortunately, there was extensive inflammation of the gingiva which followed the procedure.

Innumerable substances during this time period were used as implants; these included silver capsules, corrugated porcelain, and iridium tubes .

Radiographs taken in the 1970's of Mayan mandibles show compact bone formation around the implants-bone that amazingly looks very much like that seen around blade implants.

Dr. EJ Greenfield, in 1913, placed a "24-gauge hollow latticed cylinder of iridio-platinum soldered with 24-karat gold" as an artificial root to "fit exactly the circular incision made for it in the jaw-bone of the patient "

In the 1930's, two brothers, Drs. Alvin and Moses Strock, experimented with orthopedic screw fixtures made of Vitallium -chromium-cobalt alloy. They carefully observed how physicians successfully placed implants in the hip bone, so they implanted them in both humans and dogs to restore individual teeth.

In 1938, Dr. P.B. Adams patented a cylindrical endosseous implant that was threaded both internally and externally; it had a smooth gingival collar and a healing cap .

A post-type endosseous implant was developed by Formiggini -"Father of Modern Implantology" and Zepponi in the 1940's.

The spiral stainless steel design of the implant allowed bone to grow into the metal . This spiral implant was made by constructing a stainless steel wire on itself.
Dr. Perron Andres from Spain modified Formiggini's spiral design to include a solid shaft in the construction .

Dr. Raphael Chercheve from France added to the spiral design by creating burs to ease the insertion of the implant for a best fit. As the progression of implant discovery continued, the subperiosteal (on the bone) implant was developed in the 1940's by Dahl in Sweden. The subperiosteal implant design was further researched and elaborated upon by Lew, Bausch, and Berman in 1950.

Various implant designs expanded in the 1960's. Dr. Cherchieve crafted a double-helical spiral implant; it was made of cobalt and chromium.

In 1967, there were two variations of the blade implant that were introduced by Linkow, making it possible to place it in either the maxilla or the mandible. Linkow developed the Ventplant implant . The blade implant is now recognized as an endosseous implant.

Weiss and Judy made popular the use of intramucosal inserts during this time; the inserts helped in the retention of removable maxillary prostheses.

In 1975, an implant device placed through a submental incision and attached to the mandible was introduced by Dr. Small.
This was known as the first transosteal implant called the mandibular staple implant. This would help those individuals who had an edentulous mandible atrophic in nature.

In 1978, Dr. P. Brånemark presented a two-stage threaded titanium root-form implant; he developed and tested a system using pure titanium screws which he termed fixtures .

These were first placed in his patients in 1965 and were the first to be well-documented and the most well-maintained dental implants thus far.
Brånemark's first patient had severe deformities of the jaw and chin, congenitally missing teeth and misaligned teeth.
Four implants were inserted into the mandible. These implants integrated within a period of six months and remained in place for the next 40 years .
He found this discovery accidentally in 1952 when he was studying blood flow in rabbit femurs by placing titanium chambers in their bone.[4]

CLASSIFICATION OF MAXILLOFACIAL DEFECTS

Maxillofacial defects are classified as:

1. Congenital

2. Acquired

- Surgical (postoperative)
- Traumatical

Depending on location maxillofacial defects are classified as:

1. **Intraoral**
   - Maxillary
   - Mandibular
   - Velo-pharingeal
2. **Extra oral**
   - Auricular defects
   - Ocular defects
   - Orbital defects
   - Nasal defects
   - Lip and cheek defects

3. **Composite defects**

Most acquired maxillary defects occur due to surgical resection of tumours.

Benign lesions require a smaller resection and are easy to restore.

Whereas malignant tumours require extensive resection, which are very difficult to restore.

Common tumours of this region are:

- Epidermoid carcinoma (mostly arising from the maxillary sinus)
- Salivary gland tumors (pleomorphic adenoma, adenoid cystic carcinoma, mucoepidermoid carcinoma and adenocarcinoma)
- Malignant mesenchymal tumors (lymphoasrcoma rhabdomyosarcoma, chondreosarcoma, neurofibrosarcoma, angiosarcoma and osteosarcoma)
- Benign mesenchymal tumors (fibroma, hemangioma, angioleomyoma, angioblastoma, fibrolipoma and myxoma).

Tumors of dental origin can also occur in the palate.

Other non-neoplastic lesions like midline granuloma, Wegener's granulomatosi, Mucormyocosis, and aspergillosis may also require surgical resection in the course of treatment. One other major cause for an acquired maxillary defect is trauma. Since one cannot predict the nature and extend of the defect produced by trauma it has been discussed separately.

Types of acquired maxillary defects:

Acquired maxillary defects are usually classified based on their extent. If both the maxilla is resected, the defect is considered as total maxillectomy.

Resection of one or a part of the maxilla or palate is considered as partial maxillectomy.

Aramany proposed a classification of partial maxillary defects based on their extent.

- **Class I:** It is a unilateral defect involving one half of the arch and the adjacent palatine shelf. The defect extends to the midline -all the teeth in that side of the arch are missing (Fig 1.10).
- **Class II**: It is a unilateral defect involving one side of the arch posterior to the canine -teeth posterior to the canine are absent (Fig 1.11).
- **Class III:** It is a defect involving the center of the palatine shelves -all the teeth are present (fig 1.12).

- **Class IV:** It is a bilateral defect involving one side of the arch a long with theentire premaxilla -all anteriors along with the posteriors of one side are missing (fig 1.13).
- **Class V :** It is a bilateral posterior defect -teeth anterior to the second premolar are present (fig 1.14).
- **Class VI:** It is a bilateral anterior defects -teeth anterior to the second premolar are absent [4]

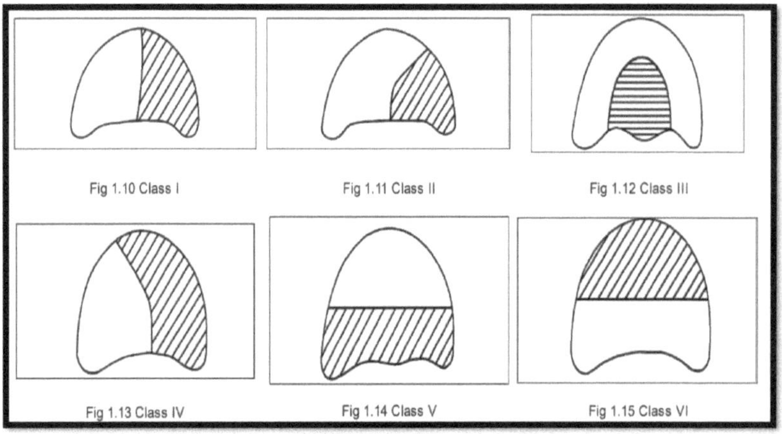

Fig 1.10 Class I
Fig 1.11 Class II
Fig 1.12 Class III
Fig 1.13 Class IV
Fig 1.14 Class V
Fig 1.15 Class VI

FIGURE: 1

MANDIBULAR DEFECTS

Congenital Defects of the Mandible Congenital mandibular defects that require a maxillofacial prosthesis are uncommon.

Common congenital defects of the mandible include

- Micrognathia
- Mandibulofacial dysostosis
- Ankylosis of the temporomandibular joint (TMJ).

Acquired Defects of the Mandible As mentioned for the maxilla, neoplastic resection is one of the most common causes for an acquired mandibular defect.

The common neoplasia which advocate the need for resection are squamous cell carcinoma of the tongue, oropharynx and floor of the mouth.[4]

These tumours are usually treated by surgery, radiation or both. Involvement of deep cervical lymph nodes is common and hence radical neck dissection is necessary. Resection of the mandible may often lead to speech and swallowing dysfunction, which are vary difficult to manage. [5]

Based on the amount of resection or bone loss (extent), mandibular defects can be classified as follows:

Continuity defect:

Here the superior portion of the mandible is resected and the lower border is left intact. The defect is located in alveolar process and integrity of mandible is preserved. These defects do not show any deviation and are easy to restore.

Discontinuity defect:

Here the entire segment of the mandible is resected. Since there is no connection between the remaining parts of the mandible, there will be midline deviation of the mandible due to the movement of the bone. Deviation may also occur when the remaining ends are surgically approximated in order to produce continuity.[5]

The amount of facial disfigurement of these defects is remarkable.

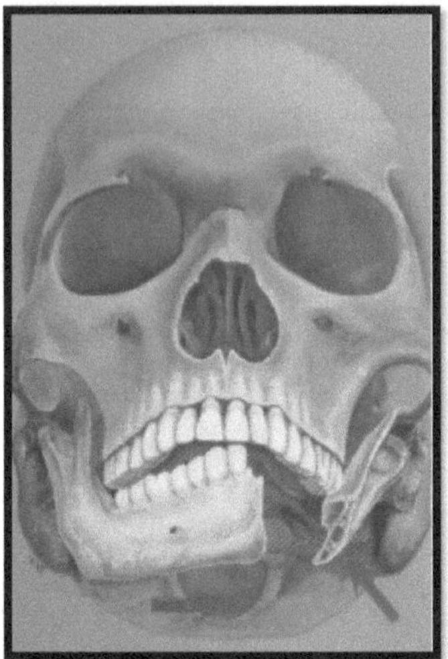

FIGURE:2

Cantor and Curtis classification of acquired mandibular defects:

• Class I: Marginal resection. Continuity defect, when the alveolar process is resected, but the lower border of the mandible is preserved .

• Class II: Segmental free end resection (discontinuity defect) that dose not cross the midline .

Modification a: Bilateral resection posterior to the second premolar.

Modification b: Unilateral resection posterior to the lateral incisor .

Modification c: Bilateral resection posterior to the lateral incisor on one side and the second premolar on the other .

• Class III: Segmental free end resection up to or crosses the midline.

• Class IV: Class III+ resection of the TMJ

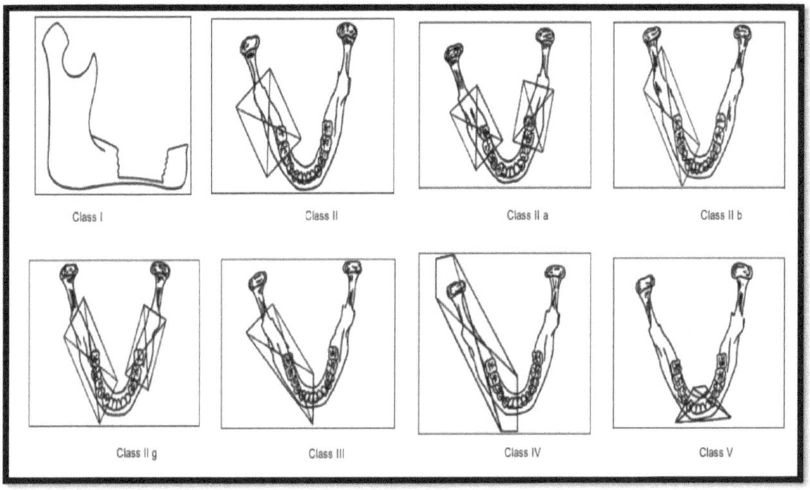

FIGURE:3a

Class V :Anterior bounded resection.[6]

Veaus classification of cleft (1931)

Group I Defects of the soft palate only .

Group II Defects involving the hard palate and soft palate .

Group III Defects involving the soft palate to the alveolus, usually involving the lip.

Group IV Complete bilateral clefts.

Liverpool Classification of Maxillectomy Defects (2000)

- Brown et al in 2000, classified surgical defects separately according to the vertical and horizontal components of the defect.[6]

The classification is as follows :

Vertical Component

Class 1: - Maxillectomy not causing oro-nasal fistula.

Class 2: - Maxillectomy not involving the orbit.

Class 3: - Maxillectomy involving the orbital adnexae with orbital retention.

Class 4: - Maxillectomy with orbital enucleation or exenteration.

Class 5: - Orbitomaxillary defect.

Class 6: - Nasomaxillary defect.

Horizontal Component

Letter a: - Palatal defect only.

Letter b: - Less than or equal to half of the bilateral maxilla.

Letter c: - Less than or equal to half of unilateral maxilla.

Letter d: -Greater than half of the maxillectomy

Durrani et al, Classification of Maxillary Defects (2013): -

Based on their research and surgical experience. Their classification is as follows:

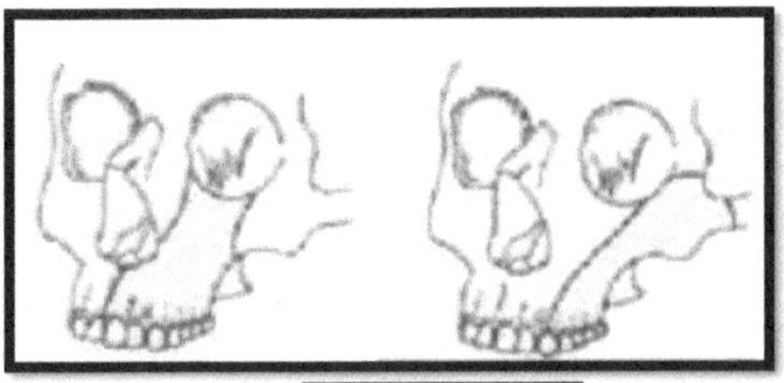

FIGURE:3B

1. Alveolectomy: - These defects involve the alveolar bone alone.

2. Sub-total Maxillectomy: - These defects cause oro-nasal or oro-antral fistula but do not disturb the orbital wall of maxilla.

3. Total Maxillectomy: - These defects are characterized by absence of complete maxilla including orbital floor but the orbital contents remain intact.

4. Radical Maxillectomy: - These defects are characterized by absence of orbital contents along with the maxilla.

5. Composite Maxillectomy: - These defects involve resection of facial skin, soft palate, and any other part of the oral cavity. All these defects can be further classified into Unilateral and Bilateral defects.[6]

RETENTION IN MAXILLOFACIAL PROSTHESIS

Any defect of the face or associated structures may be congenital or acquired.

Congenital defects are the defects or malformations present from birth whereas the acquired defects may be due to accidents, gunshot injuries, cancer treatment, ablative surgery and animal bite.

These malformations affect the well-being of the individual affecting them psychologically depriving the confidence levels.

So the reconstruction of these lost or malformed structures is essential.

Maxillofacial defect reconstruction can be made by three ways:

1. Surgical reconstruction by alloplastic or autogenous grafts
2. Maxillofacial or craniofacial prosthesis rehabilitation.
3. Combination of the above two.[7]

Reconstruction of facial defects is a complex modality either surgically or prosthetically driven depending on the site, size, etiology, severity, age and the expectation of the patient.

Whenever surgical reconstruction is not possible or failure of the alloplastic or autogenous graft occurs, maxillofacial or craniofacial prosthesis becomes an alternative method. [8]

RETENTIVE MECHANISM

Maxillofacial prosthesis is retained through various methods for their retention and support.

Each retentive mechanism is having its own advantage and disadvantage.

The various retentive aids available are :

1) Adhesive

2) Skin tapes/ straps/ suture material/toupee tapes.

3) Spectacle frames

4) Soft tissue or bony undercuts, anatomic projections using them as mechanical interlocks

5) Implants.

These retentive aids are selected based on the various factors such as the extent of prosthesis, availability of bone, radiation therapy, patient's dexterity, location, amount of hard and soft tissue available and compliance of the patient.[7]

Magnets or clips can be used to effectively retain the prostheses and will also minimize force transfer to the implant and supporting bone. The resultant decrease in dependence on chemical (adhesives) and anatomic (tissue undercuts) retention is beneficial to both the patient and the prosthodontist.[8]

Cast clasps: The most common method for retaining an intraoral prosthesis uses a cast metal clasp which enters an undercut.

The properly designed and fabricated clasp will provide stability, splinting, bilateral bracing, and reciprocation, as well as retention. Retainers are probably the most important components contributing to the success of the obturator prosthesis.

It helps in favorable load distribution and also help in retention of prosthesis.

Acrylic buttons: Acrylic buttons retained facial prostheses usually have an acrylic substructure that fits into the defect and one or more mushroom - shaped acrylic projections (buttons) attached to the substructure. The final prosthesis is fabricated so that it will snap over the mushroom buttons for retention.[7]

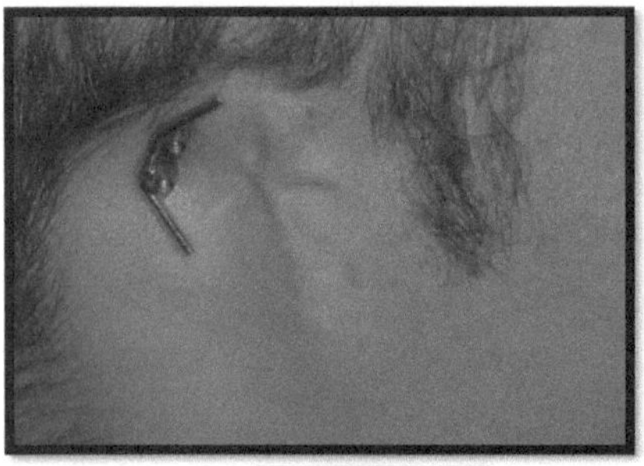

FIGURE: 4

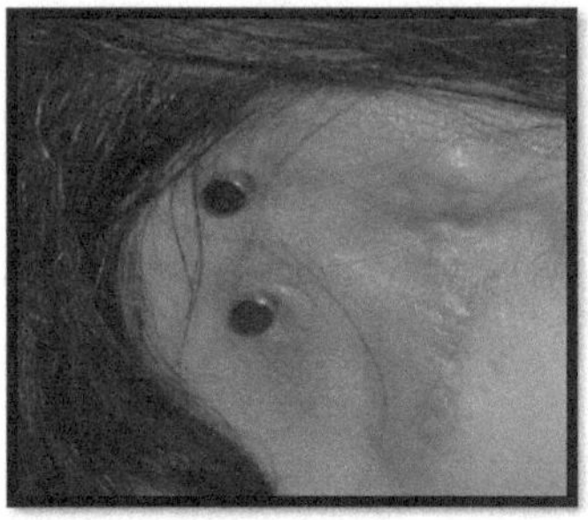

FIGURE: 5

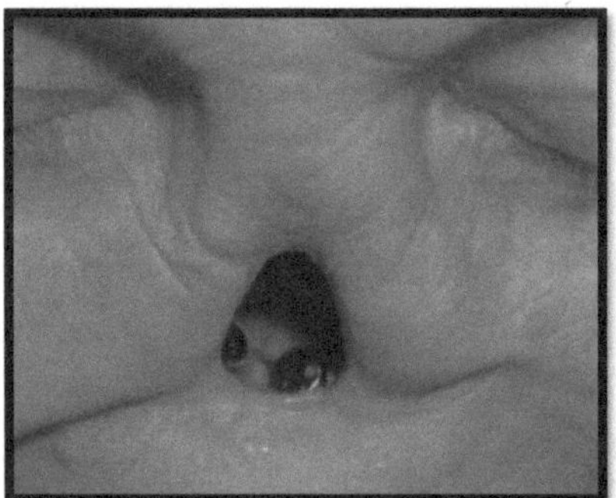

FIGURE:6

Fig 4, 5, 6 :Different retention options for attachment of maxillofacial prostheses

Biomechanical Considerations Of Implants In Maxillofacial Prosthesis:

a) Design of craniofacial and intraoral implant:-

Craniofacial implants are less diverse than intraoral implants. They are available in smaller lengths of 3-4mm as the availability of bone is limited.

It has a flange with perforations which increases surface area enhancing initial mechanical stability of implant design during healing period and also help prevent tilting of the implant under the action of lateral forces and moments.

b) Micromotion at the Bone-Implant Interface:-

Implants placed should be relatively immobile in order to have enhanced osseointegration.

Any micromotion in such site causes formation of fibrous tissues leading to failure in osseointegration.

c) Stress Transfer from implants to bone:-

Implants should never be stressed beyond their loading capacity.

Unlike intraoral implants which are stressed 50-200N craniofacial implants are stressed 0.1 – 1N.

The designing of implant screw transmit an axial tensile or compressive load to the surrounding bone, primarily by compression on the inclined faces of the screw.

d) Load distribution to several screws:-

When prosthesis is supported by several screws, the resulting combined structure forms a unit in which the distribution of any applied load is distributed evenly among all the members involved, which depends on the relative stiffness and geometry of their arrangement.

e) Impact of implant stiffness on stress distribution:-

Stiffness of implant depends on the diameter of the implant. If the diameter is increased by 30%, implant stiffness will be five times higher, and the stresses around the implant neck are thus reduced dramatically.

f) Impact of the implant shape on stress distribution:-

The stress conditions around an implant can also be improved by selecting an appropriate implant shape .

Because force transfer into bone should be as even as possible, implants showing rational symmetry can be considered more favourable for stress distribution

g) Impact of the implant surface on stress distribution:-

The implant surface used for force transfer should be as large as possible.

To minimize the compressive forces, the implant surface can be enlarged by applying threads or by plasma flame spray coating or surface roughening and acid etching.

h) Measurement of implant stability and Osseointegration:-

Methods to evaluate implant stability are histological analysis, percussion tests, reverse and vibration tests (perio test and radiofrequency analysis test). In radiofrequency analysis technique evaluates bone quality at the time of implant placement and changes in stiffness at the implant tissue interface attributable to bone formation during healing. There is decrease in resonance frequency and an increase in damping if an implant fails to integrate because of fibrous tissue formation at the interface.[9]

OSSEOINTEGRATION

It is necessary to have a clear concept about the science of implantation and the healing of bone following a successful implant placement.

Osseous healing along an implant follows a similar process to fracture healing but is subjective to the nature of the surface of the implant .

As soon as blood comes into contact with the surface of the implant, proteins adsorb to it, platelets get activated and bind to the adsorbed protein which results in the formation of a clot.

This coagulum at the implant surface supports the deposition of proteins, releases inflammatory mediators and initiates new tissue formation.

The release of numerous signaling molecules influence the migration of monocytes, neutrophils (both involved in inflammation), and mesenchymal cells (cells that can differentiate into osteoblasts) towards the implant surface.

Following the aggregation of neutrophils and macrophages from nearby capillary beds to the implant site there is further release of inflammatory mediators which are necessary for the initiation of osteogenesis.

Components of tissue growth factor β (TGF-β) super-family are also expressed within 24 hours of implantation, including bone morphogenetic proteins (BMPs) and growth & differentiation factors (GDFs).

These signaling molecules result in the collection, migration, and differentiation of mesenchymal cells, which take part in the formation of woven bone.

Woven bone subsequently undergoes a sequence of remodeling, resulting in the formation of mature bone which is the desired end result .

Factors of importance for predictable osseointegration

There are six factors of importance that must be carefully monitored to ensure predictable osseointegration.

Material of the fixture-Titanium alloys are the most commonly used as these are known to integrate in the bone without causing adverse effects. It can remain incorporated into the bone for many decades, and be used as anchorage for different prostheses.

Macrostructure of the implant-A screw-shaped implant ensures better primary stability as compared to a conical shaped implant. This may be due to micro-movements of the conical shape and reduced osseointegration.

Microstructure of the implant-Original Brånemark implants had a smooth surface as they were manufactured by machining. Clinically however it has been observed that very smooth surfaces have lesser degree of osseointegration, along with minor amount of resorption. On the other hand a highly roughened surface shows rapid integration; but later secondary inflammation and secondary resorption is noticed that can endanger the long-term survival of the implant.

Osseous bed into which the implant is placed-Geriatric patients with bone that is osteoporotic will show lesser degree of osseointegration. Similar is the case of patients who have had radiotherapy or who have sustained severe burns that alter the osseous quality and reduce its capacity for osseointegration.

Surgical technique – The surgical intervention should be carefully monitored with slow speed, high torque and copious irrigation with cold water.The temperature should never be allowed to rise as the osteoblasts are extremely heat labile and get damaged easily. The implant itself should never be touched by gloves or gauze. It is vital that the surgical bed be free from fibers, powder and any other foreign matter that might hinder osseointegration.

Loading the implant – The implant should be loaded along its long axis as far as feasible. Lateral, torsional or cantilever forces are least tolerated and should be minimized by efficient planning and design.

Extraoral implant systems:-

There are 2 systems available, solitary and grouped.

In solitary systems single implants are available whereas in grouped implants, grid or plate systems are present which are secured by several screws.

Extraoral implants with solitary systems are Branemark systems, ITI systems, IMZ system, ankylose system, southern implants and epiplant system. Grouped implant systems are epitec and epiplating systems.[10]

Features of extraoral implants:-

Generally four types of thread forms are suggested for implants - V-form, square, buttress and reverse buttress.

Out of these, V- form is most commonly used as endosseous intraoral implant.

Though square thread is able to transmit high compressive and low shear forces to bone, it is unsuitable for small implant length.

Buttress thread form are considered as more suitable for supporting maxillofacial prosthesis.

During routine removal and reinsertion of the prosthesis, tensile and compressive forces acts on the implant.

Compressive stresses are effectively resisted by bone whereas the tensile forces may prove detrimental to the implant survival. Reverse buttress thread form can take care of the pull out force to a greater extent because the outward thread face is flat.

So reverse buttress thread forms can also be used in supporting the maxillofacial prosthesis.[11]

In contrast to intraoral implants which are available in market with wide range of shapes, designs and surface modifications extraoral implants are less diverse.
These are comparatively shorter in length and have a dual structure with an endosseous part and a thread in abutment. [10]

Generally a perforated flange is provided to increase the implant surface area to have more bone to implant contact (BIC) to facilitate initial immobilization and prevent undue intracranial pressure.

Various maxillofacial or craniofacial prosthesis retained by extraoral implants are ear prosthesis, auricular prosthesis, orbital prosthesis and finger prosthesis.
To place an extraoral implant, fabrication of a surgical template is necessary or prerequisite.

It helps in pre-treatment planning by determining the oriental position and location of the Implant.
These surgical templates can be designed and fabricated either manually or digitally.[11]

Craniofacial Implant Classification:-

Based on the amount of bone available for the placement of implant fixtures craniofacial implants are classified as;

(1) Alpha

(2) Beta and

(3) Gamma sites

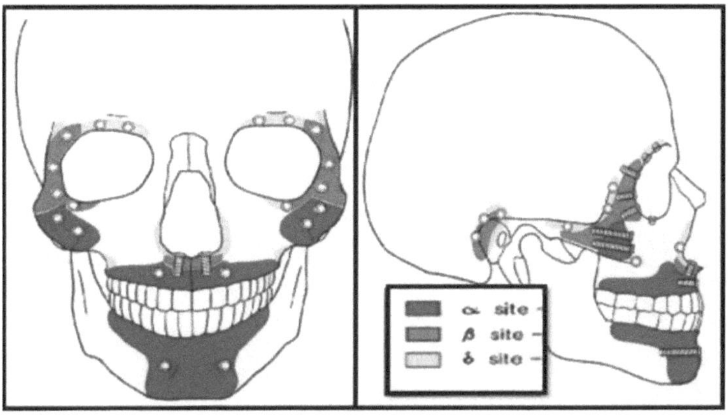

FIGURE:7

Alpha sites:

- In these sites amount of bone available is more ranging from 6mm or greater.
- Can withstand greater loads and regular fixtures.
- These may be used to retain complex facial prosthesis or dental prosthesis.
- Zygoma, anterior maxilla and mandible are the alpha sites in craniofacial region.

Beta sites:

- These are found in the periorbital but also in the temporal, zygomatic, and anterior nasal fossa locations.
- These use short dental fixtures (5mm)or phalanged fixtures (4mm).

Delta sites:

- Includes the buttress, pyriform zygomatic arch, medial orbit, temporal and frontal bones, and zygomatico-frontal process.
- Implant fixtures used are 3mm or less.[12]

IMPLANT SYSTEMS IN MAXILOFACIAL PROSTHESIS

There are 2 systems available, **solitary and grouped**.

- In solitary systems single implants are available whereas in grouped implants, grid or plate systems are present which are secured by several screws. [13]

Extraoral implants with solitary systems are :

1) **Branemark systems**
2) **ITI systems**
3) **IMZ system**
4) **Ankylose system**
5) **Southern implants**
6) **Epiplant system.**

- Grouped implant systems are **epitec and epiplating** systems.

I. BRANEMARK SYSTEM (VISTAFIX)

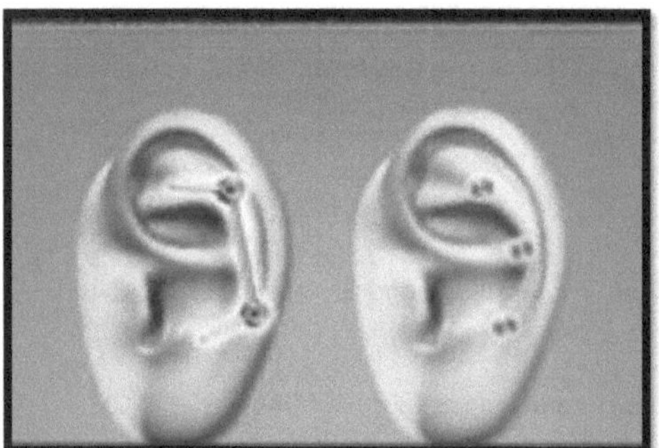

FIGURE:8

- First implant system to be used extraorally.
- For the extraoral area, titanium screws of a length of 3 and 4 mm (and 5.5 mm) are available.
- Closed flange or flangeless implants are used to avoid trauma.
- Special clamps are given for abutment.

II. ITI SYSTEMS

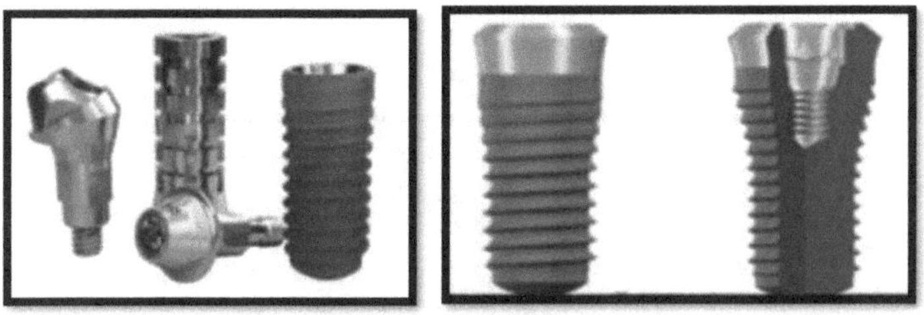

FIGURE:9

- International team for implantology.
- Sand blasted, large grit, acid etched surface(SLA).
- Two staged roughness.
- For the extraoral region ,self-tapping titanium screws with a diameter of 3.3 mm and a countersunk depth of 3.5 or 5 mm with a coned seat are used.[13]

GROUPED IMPLANTS

- In 1956, Köle and Wirth described subperiosteal frame implants made of Wisil® , a cobalt chrome alloy.

- These subperiosteal implants were adapted to the bone surface, without being anchored into the bone itself.
- The prosthesis attachment takes place on parts of the frame implant projecting through the skin.
- In contrast to the **solitary implants**, the forces are distributed across the plate over several titanium bone screws.

- An already thinned out area can be used again following the loss of another (solitary) implant.
- In this way a **secure fixing in anatomically difficult regions with limited bone area** is possible.

III. EPITEC SYSTEM

- By Mostafa farmand and leibinger company (1991).
- This system consists of a 3D carrier plate and self tapping 2mm titanium screws.

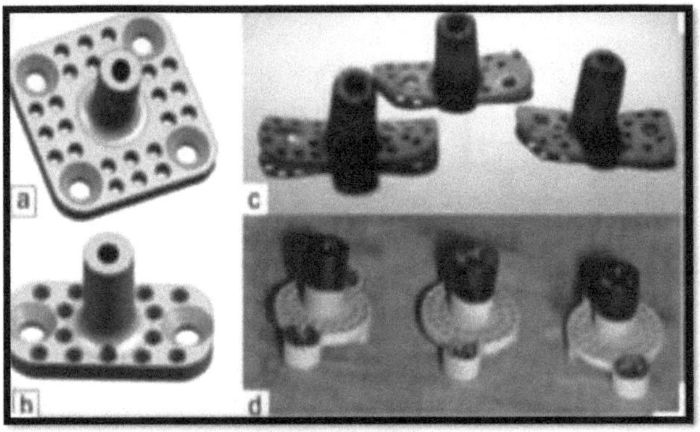

FIGURE:10

IV.EPIPLATING SYSTEM

- Given by Federspil and M. Schneider (2000).
- The titanium plates of the Epiplating system are 1 mm thick, but 2 mm in width and are thus stronger than the Epitec grid system.
- To anchor the plates , titanium with screws of 2mm in breadth and lengths of:4, 5.5 and 7mm are used.
- The plates are more resistant against rotational forces which occur when screwing down and unscrewing the mountings.[14]

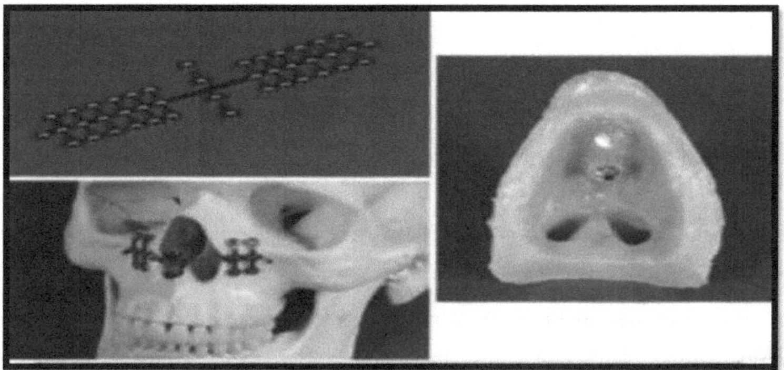

FIGURE:11

INTRAORAL IMPLANTS

1. **Basal Implants:**

Basal implantology also termed bi-cortical implantology, cortical implantology and strategic implantology.

Cortico-Basal Implantology® is a modern innovative implantology system which utilizes the basal cortical portion of the jaw bones for retention of the dental implants, which are less prone to resorption and are infection free.

Originally, dental implants were considered as "last resort" for treatment of the edentulous patients. [14]

As implant dentistry progressed, the original Brånemark protocol required long healing periods of several months for osseointegration to take place before beginning fabrication of the definitive prosthesis.

Dentists consequently became profoundly aware of time-dependent relationship between form and functional changes in the masticatory system.

Such knowledge helped nurture the development of new materials and knowledge about the relationships between esthetics, occlusion, and patient's personalities.

Basal bone is defined as the osseous tissue of the mandible and maxilla other than the alveolar processes.

It acts as the basic framework of the maxilla and mandible.

The basal bone is always present throughout life; it is very strong and forms the stress-bearing part of our skeleton.

Utilizing the basal bone, implantologists can now place implants in regions where traditional implants would not be possible.

Basal implants have unique design and are available in various types.

Crestal basal implants, one among the type of basal implants, are placed flapless with no incision required.

They engage the second or third cortical plates for which osseointegration is not paramount.

The term "osseointegration" is called "osseoadaptation" by basal implantologist, this stems from the fact that the bone with continuous functional loads remodels and adapts over the implant surface.[7]

A. Indications:

a. Patients presented with partial or full edentulism in the upper or lower jaw

b. Patients having atrophied ridges.

c. Patients in whom placement of conventional implants would result in poor prognosis due to various reasons.

d. Patients with failed bone augmentation procedures.

B. Contraindications:

1. Any systemic condition which contradicts any surgical procedure
2. If suspected that the treatment could affect the patient's health condition like pregnancy .
3. Any patient on IV bisphosphonate therapy

4. The planned implant area having persisting lesions, such as a tumour, or showed signs of chronic bone diseases which may continue even after implant placement

5. History of radiotherapy in the head-and-neck region for malignancies, chemotherapy for treatment of malignancy within 1 year of the procedure desired

6. If the patient's cooperation appeared questionable

7. If the patient did not give his or her informed consent to participate. [14]

In general, on a patient, if a routine simple extraction can be done, full-mouth rehabilitation with strategic implantology can be routinely done.[14]

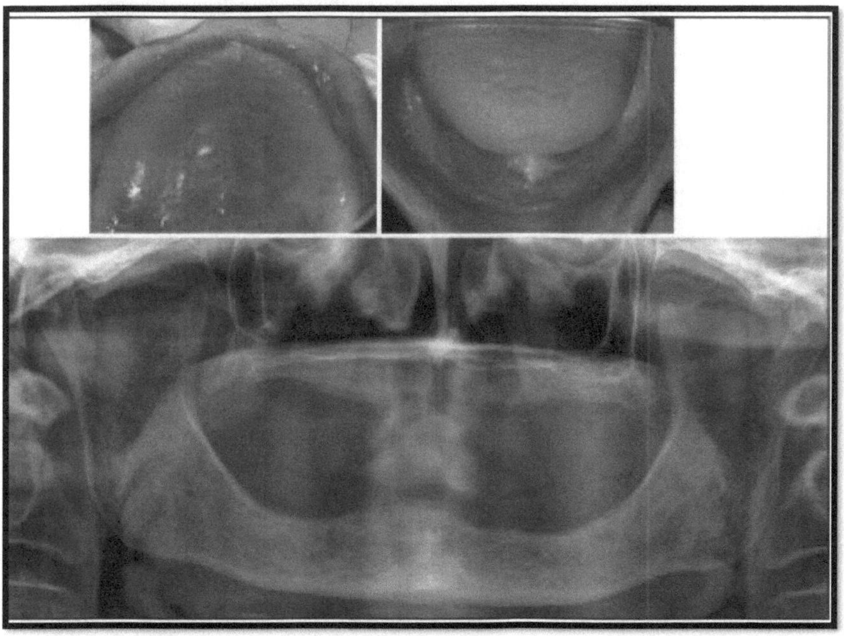

FIGURE:12

Preoperative orthopantomogram and clinical photograph

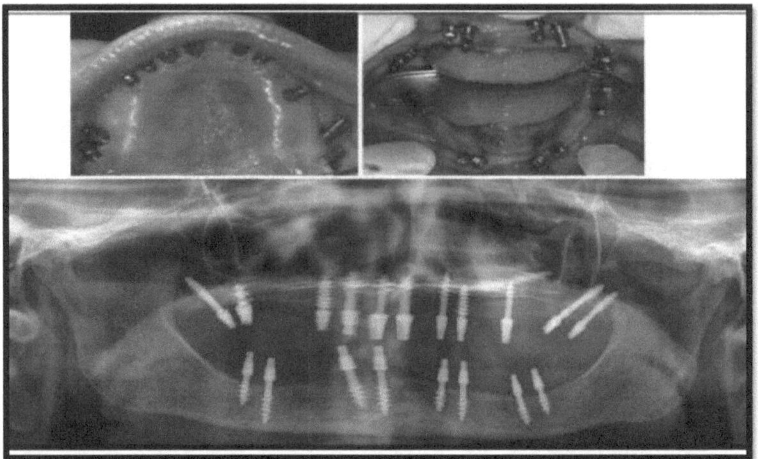

FIGURE:13

Intraoperative orthopantomogram and clinical photograph

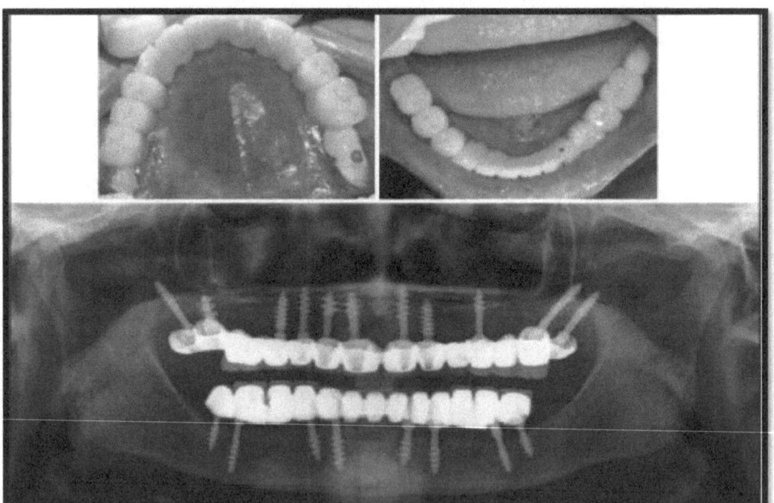

FIGURE:14

Postoperative orthopantomogram and clinical photograph.

Intraoperative procedures included extraction, curettage, implant placement, and impression making.

The procedure of implant placement was performed under local anesthetic solution 2% lignocaine with adrenaline in 1:80,000 dilution by giving infiltration and field block.

Nerve blocks were completely avoided during the procedure to judge the proximity to vital anatomical structures and to avoid accidental insertion of implants at critical positions.

After implant placement, impression was made by additional silicon putty and master cast was readied on the same day after recording jaw relation.

Postoperatively, 2 ml dexona was injected intraorally and the patient was prescribed analgesics tablet paracetamol 500 mg + aceclofenac 100 mg BD for 3–5 days.

Necessary instructions of diet and oral hygiene were given.

On the next day (2nd day) of implant placement, metal framework try-in made up of Co-Cr metal was taken up.

Various adjustments regarding the height, width, and angulation were done on implants using metal cutting bur such that the metal framework snuggly fits over the implants.

Teeth selection and shade selection procedure for prosthesis was also performed.

For patients in whom excessive shrinkage was expected due to inflamed tissue, hybrid prosthesis was preferred as interim prosthesis and the patient was explained about the need for replacement of prosthesis later on, whereas ceramic veneered circular bridges were preferred for most cases.

On the next day of metal try-in (3rd day), either final prosthesis consisting of metal frame and veneering from either ceramics or acrylic was cemented by using glass-ionomer cement after final bite adjustment.[15]

2. **SUBPERIOSTEAL IMPLANTS:**

The **subperiosteal implant** consists of a metal framework that is custom fitted to the patient's jaw or jaw bone and gum tissue.

The metal framework is placed over the bone and held in place with small metal posts that penetrate through the gum and into the underlying bone.

As the gum tissue heals, it adheres to the metal framework and helps hold it in place.

Once the **subperiosteal implant** has been securely attached to the bone, artificial teeth can be attached to the metal posts.
These teeth can be removable or fixed, depending on the needs and preferences of the patient.

Used when:

- Subperiosteal implants are often used for patients who have experienced significant resorption or thinning of the maxillary or mandibular bone as a result of injury, periodontal disease, aging, or other factors.

- They are also commonly used for patients who are not good candidates for bone grafting procedures .

- Who prefer to avoid the time and cost associated with these procedures.[16]

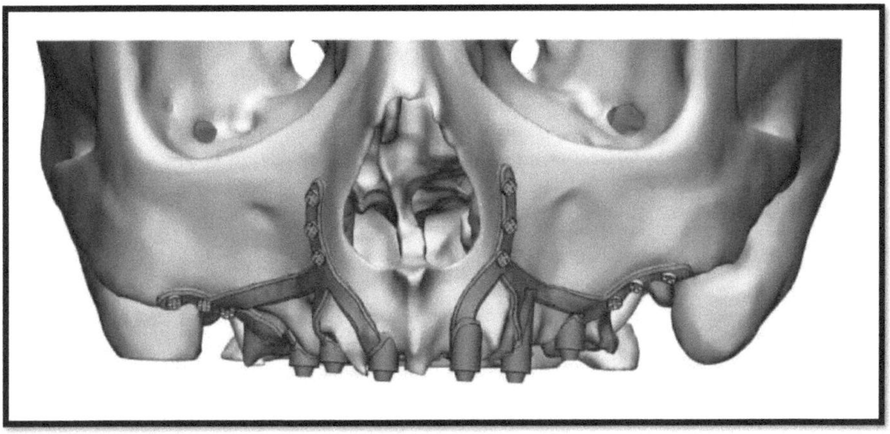

FIGURE:15

ADVANTAGES:

- **No Bone Grafting Required**: Subperiosteal implants don't require bone grafting procedures before placement, making the process quicker and less invasive.
- **Suitable for Patients With Insufficient Jawbone Density**: These dental implants work well for patients with insufficient jawbone density who may not be candidates for traditional endosteal dental implants.
- **Stable and Durable**: They're anchored to the jawbone using small posts, providing a stable and durable foundation for replacement teeth.
- **Customizable**: These implants can be custom-made and attached to the patient's jaw, ensuring a comfortable and natural-looking fit.
- **Versatile**: Subperiosteal implants can be used to replace one or multiple missing teeth or support a full arch restoration or full mouth rehabilitation.
- **Easy to Clean and Maintain**: They can be cleaned just like natural teeth, making it easy for patients to maintain good oral hygiene.

DISADVANTAGES:

- **Invasive Surgery**: The procedure for a subperiosteal implant is more invasive than other types of implants, such as endosteal implants. This can result in more pain, an increased risk of complications, and a longer recovery time for patients.
- **Risk of Infection**: Since the implant is placed under the gum tissue, there's a higher risk of infection. This can be especially problematic if the implant becomes loose or shifts, as it can create a pocket where bacteria can accumulate.
- **Limited Placement**: Subperiosteal implants are not suitable for all patients. They're typically only used in cases where there's not enough bone to support the implant. However, even in these cases, not all patients are good candidates for a subperiosteal implant.
- **Cost**: Subperiosteal implants can be more expensive than other types, as they require more complex surgical procedures and custom fabrication.
- **Limited Long-Term Data**: While subperiosteal implants have been used for many years, there's still limited long-term data on their effectiveness and longevity. This means that it may be difficult to predict how well they will perform over time.[16]

Why Subperiosteal Implants Are Rarely Used Today?

Despite the advantages of subperiosteal implants, they're rarely used today compared to traditional endosteal implants or even zygomatic implants.

The main reason is the advancements in bone grafting procedures, which have made it possible for patients with insufficient jawbone density to undergo a bone grafting procedure and receive a traditional endosteal implant.

Also, a subperiosteal implant requires a metal frame to be anchored to the jawbone, which can sometimes cause discomfort and make it difficult to clean the implant effectively. This can increase the risk of infection and may lead to implant failure over time.

In addition, subperiosteal implants are generally more complex and time-consuming to place compared to endosteal implants and require a higher level of expertise and skill from the dentist. As a result, not all dentists are trained to place subperiosteal implants, and patients may need to travel to a specialist center to receive this implant.

In recent years, advancements in dental implant technology have resulted in the development of alternative implant treatments that are less invasive and provide similar benefits to subperiosteal implants. These new implant systems are now widely available and are often a preferred option for patients who require dental implant treatment.[17]

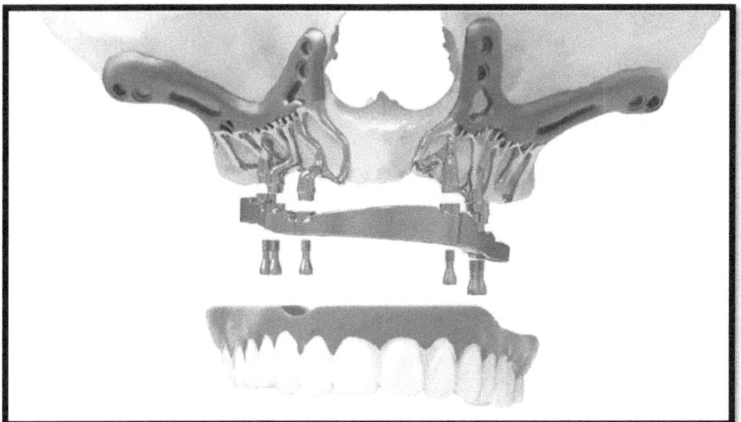

FIGURE:16

3. ZYGOMATIC IMPLANTS:

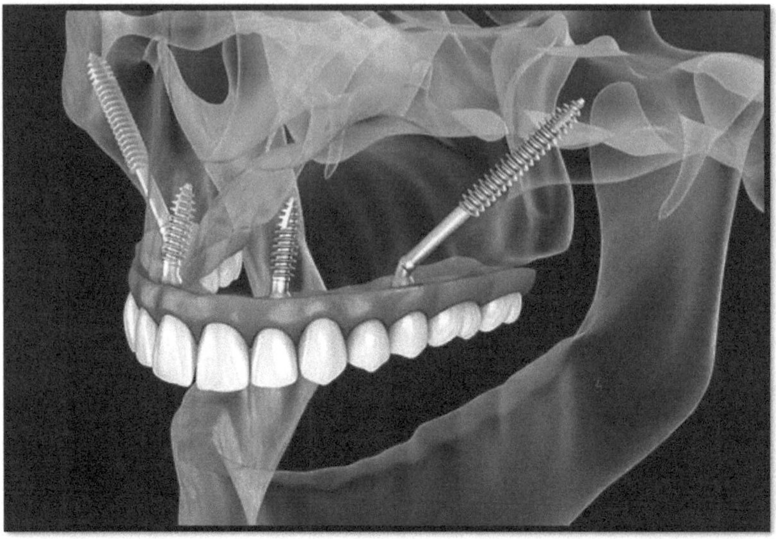

FIGURE:17

Zygomatic implant (ZI) therapy is an elective treatment modality for the rehabilitation of partially and fully edentulous patients, pioneered by Branemark et al. in 1998.

It was proposed that zygomatic implants are an evidence-based surgical and prosthetic solution for both two-stage and immediate loading protocols, using either intra-sinus or extra-sinus approaches .[18]

Their use is widespread, ranging from trauma and oral cancer rehabilitation cases to failed conventional implant cases, an alternative to augmentation in the atrophic maxilla and failed augmentation.

The need for zygomatic implants arises from the impossibility of placing regular implants due to the lack of adequate residual bone.

Indeed, zygomatic implants offer a definitive solution to lack of bone by allowing the placement of implants into zygomatic bone to anchor full arch prostheses.

The treatment of severe maxillary atrophy with zygomatic implants is a solution that enables the delivery of an immediate provisional prosthesis within 24 h of surgery.[19]

The zygomatic implant (ZI) positioning avoids the maxillary sinus lifts of onlay block grafting, which are indicated when reconstructing the severely atrophic maxilla with autologous grafts harvested from:

- Iliac crest
- Calvaria
- Intra-orally from the mandible.

Zygomatic implant surgery generally results in less severe symptoms or morbidity when compared with grafting options, which result in higher surgical morbidity, with reduced predictability, higher treatment costs and prolonged overall duration of treatment.

The zygomatic bone articulates with :

- sphenoid bone
- maxilla
- frontal bone
- temporal bone

to form the lateral wall of the floor of the orbit and contributes to the formation of the temporal and infratemporal fossa bilaterally.

Characterized by trabecular and cortical components that are ideally positioned to provide robust anchorage points for zygomatic implants.[18]

The ORIS criteria is a refined version of the Zygomatic Success Code, including four dimensions in the definition of success:

- Offset measurement as an evaluation of prosthetic positioning
- Rhino-sinus status report based on a comparison of presurgical and postsurgical cone-beam computed tomography and a clinical questionnaire.
- Infection permanence as an evaluation of soft tissue status.
- Stability report, accepting as success some mobility until dis-osseointegration signs appear.[20]

Zygomatic implant indications include severe maxillary atrophy as well as oncology reconstruction. The type of procedure studied may include between 1 and 4 zygomatic implants.

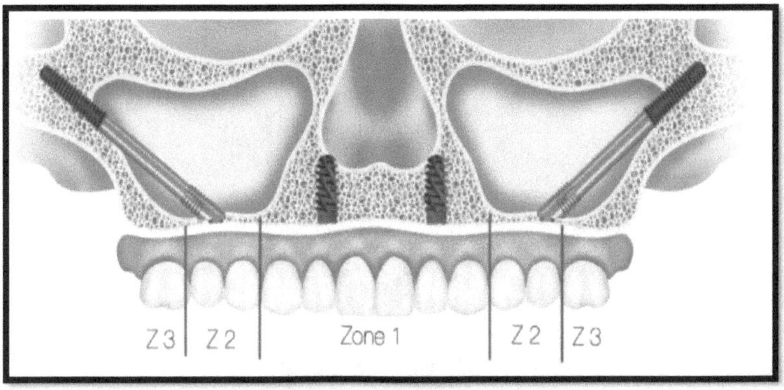

FIGURE:18

Zones of maxilla determine the indication for the zygoma concept

The zygoma implant developed by Branemark was specifically designed to offer maximum bone anchorage while simplifying access to the implant head, facilitating the abutment connection.

The zygoma implant is available in 8 lengths ranging from 30 to 52.5 mm.

The head of the zygoma implant is engineered to allow prosthesis attachment at a 45-degree angle to the long axis of the implant.

With this specific design, these implants have been successfully used to support prostheses in the atrophic edentulous maxilla as well as patients who have undergone maxillectomy.[19]

The case shown below shows defect that extends from the palatal midline to the distal surface of the left incisor and posteriorly onto the soft palate.

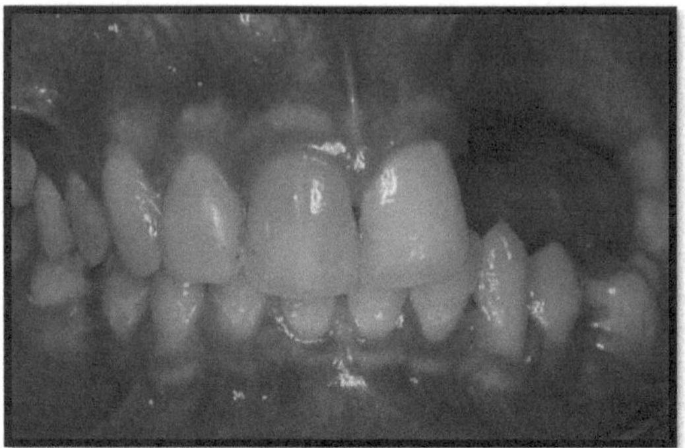

Preoperative situation

FIGURE:19

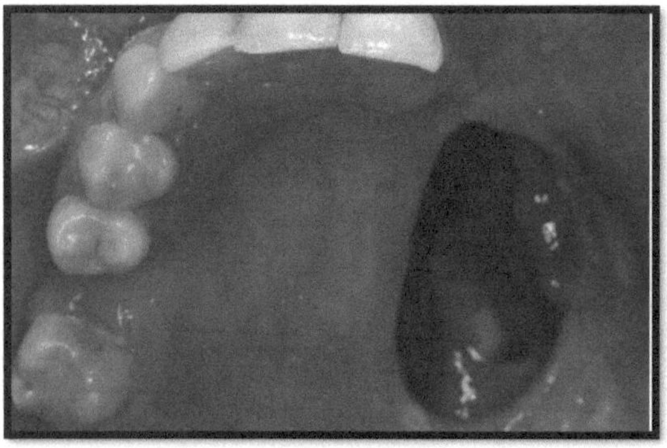

Preoperative situation

FIGURE:20

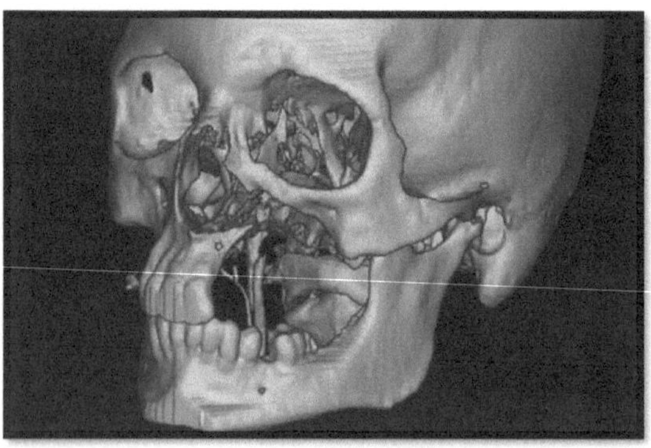

CT reconstruction showing extent of resection.

FIGURE:21

For this patient, there was no alternative to prosthetic obturation, as microsurgical rehabilitation was not considered a viable option due to the compromised vascular supply to the defect site.

Considering **stability, retention, load distribution, and suprastructure longevity**, the decision was made to rehabilitate the patient with a telescopic crown–retained obturator prosthesis, additionally supported by 1 or 2 zygoma implants (Zygomaticus Fixture; Nobel Biocare) on the defect side.

To ensure proper position and bone anchorage, navigation during the implant placement was planned.[20]

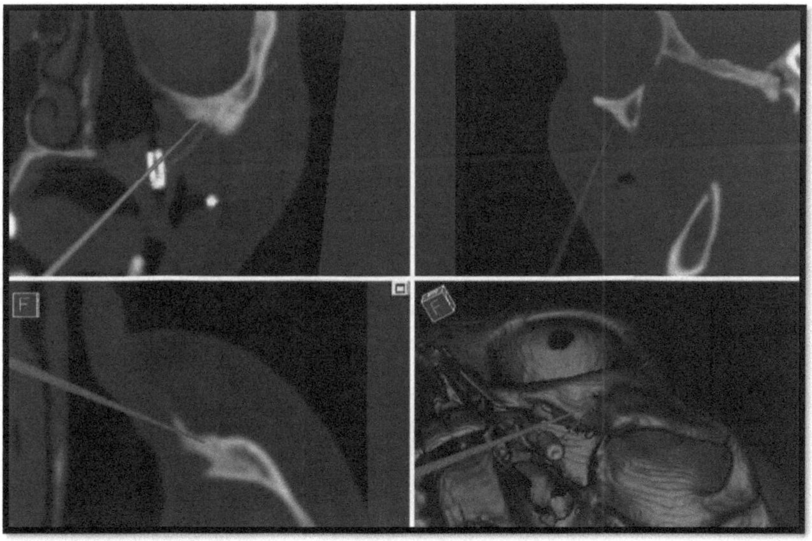

Intraoperative navigation program. Drilling direction is visible in CT in 3 different planes (upper left - frontal plane, lower left - coronal plane, upper right - sagittal plane)

FIGURE:22

After preliminary impressions with irreversible hydrocolloid, artificial teeth were diagnostically arranged on a trial basis of the maxillary prosthesis.

Using this arrangement, an acrylic resin (Probase; Ivoclar Vivadent,)template for the computed tomography (CT) was generated and a radiopaque marker (5-mm titanium drilling sleeve;) was positioned where the implant-prosthesis connection would ideally be located.

The marker was positioned so that it would not interfere with the palatal contours of the prosthesis or with the buccal flange, which was necessary for a good seal.

This information was transferred to the CT and enabled a generation of a CT-based virtual model with visualization of the ideal position of implant head using a special navigation system .

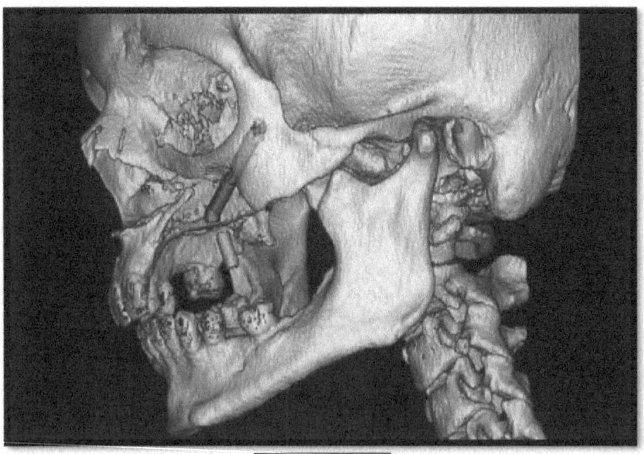

FIGURE:23

Postoperative CT scan with acrylic resin template in position. Implant head is ideally situated above marker (yellow) of template. Position and angulation of implant in zygoma bone provide sufficient anchorage.[18]

It was possible to preoperatively simulate and predetermine the ideal implant position in a 3-dimensional (3-D) reconstruction.

It became evident that it would not be possible to properly place 2 zygoma implants side by side, as the zygomatic bone was very thin in the caudal area, thus allowing the placement of only 1 implant in the thicker cranial portion.

During the 3-month healing period, all remaining teeth were prepared for a telescopic crown–retained prosthesis. [21]

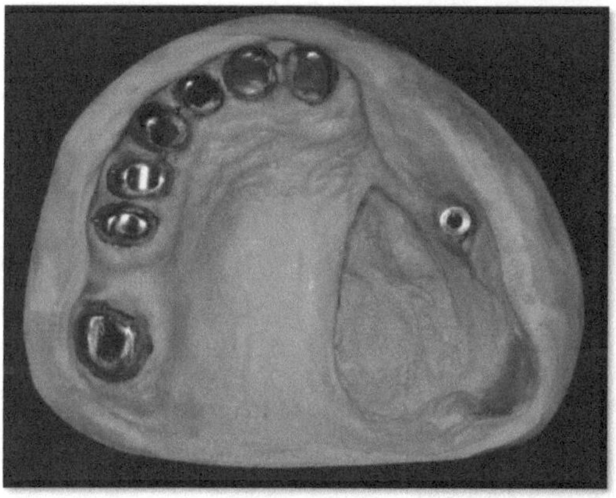

Primary crowns on definitive cast.

FIGURE:24

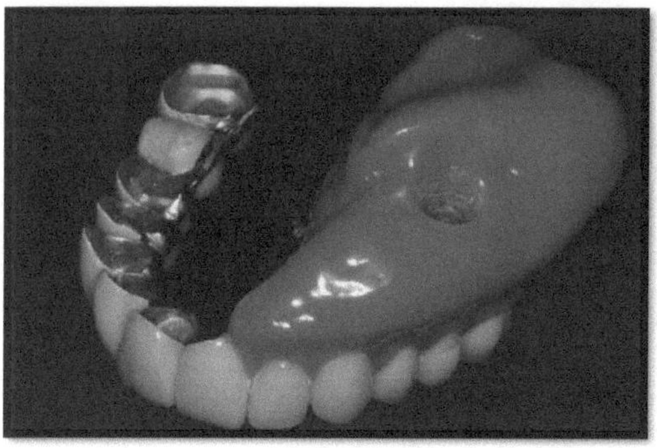

Definitive prosthesis

FIGURE:25

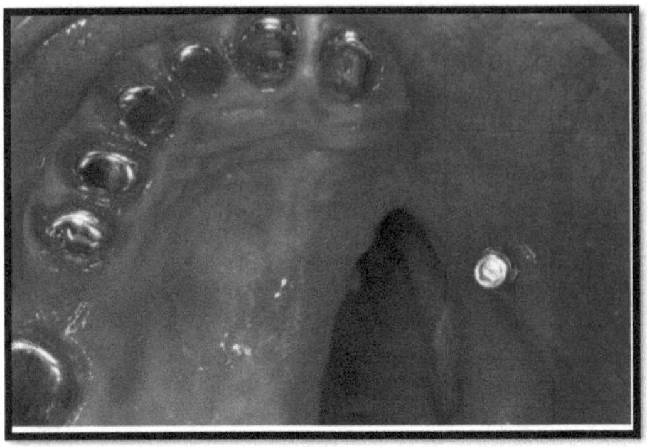

Inner telescopic crown copings after cementation.

FIGURE:26

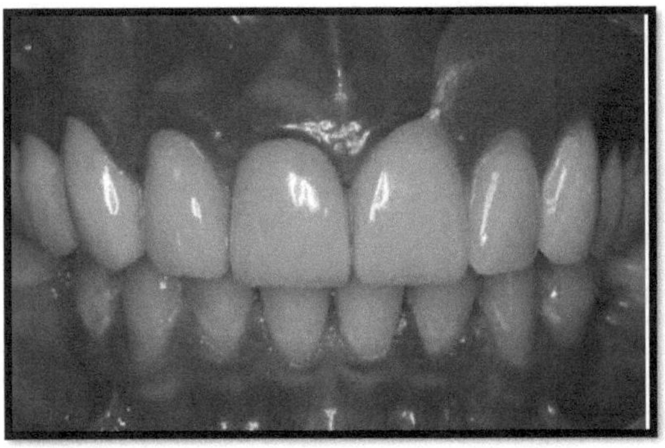

Definitive prosthesis in place

FIGURE:27

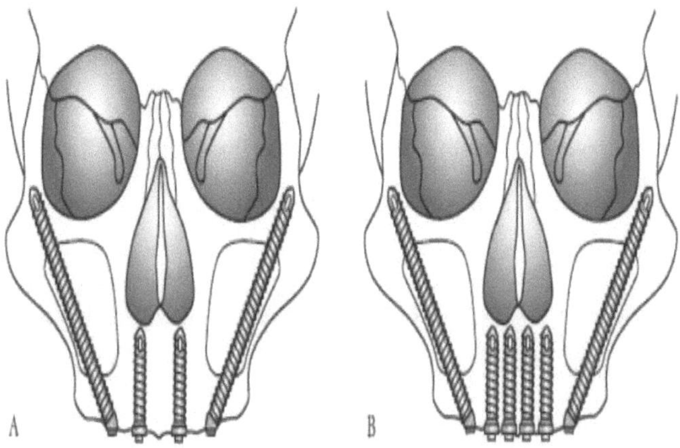

A. Pictorial representation of recommended zygoma and standard implant fixtures cross-arch stabilization and fixed restoration. B. Diagramatic representation of zygoma and implant fixtures for restoration with cross-arch stabilization and fixed restoration.

FIGURE:28

MANAGEMENT OF EDENTULOUS MAXILLECTOMY PATIENT

Edentulous maxillectomy patients are always a challenge for the maxillofacial team due to the complexity of postoperative rehabilitation.

Retention of the obturator is a problem since there is a lack of support of adjacent teeth for stabilization.

In addition, the reduced volume of residual ridge of the edentulous patient demands that stress be distributed to all available portions of the palate.[22]

Some of the important guidelines to be informed to the maxillofacial surgeon or oncosurgeon at the time of resection are as follow:

Maintain as much hard palate as possible: Since the edentulous patient must rely on remnants of the hard palate for primary retention, support and stability, the prosthodontist should advise the surgeon to resect only that portion of the hard palate that is mandatory to allow for clean margins.

It is vital to ensure that the ipsilateral palate is preserved which will allow a tripoding effect. If the anterior alveolus can be maintained, the patient will have better facial esthetics and less contracture postoperatively.

Skin graft the cheek flap :The edentulous patient requires maximal distribution of forces, and the mucosa on the cheek will be an area of contact with the obturator. The thick squamous epithelium of a split-thickness skin graft will resist the wear and tear applied by the obturator as compared to the friable oral tissues.

Remove the inferior turbinate: By removing the inferior turbinate, the prosthesis can be contoured to fit into the nasal cavity. This vertical height will resist the rotational forces applied during mastication. In addition, by adding an extension into the nasal cavity, a larger surface of bone may be utilized to balance the stresses generated during mastication.

Skin graft the maxillary sinus walls :This is necessary as the movements of the obturator bulb will transmit greater force to the sinus walls in the edentulous patient. These walls can be prepared during surgery to allow the bony undercuts to serve for retention or for vertical support to keep the prosthesis from rotating into the defect during mastication.The sinus walls are covered with respiratory mucosa, which must be denuded and covered with a split-thickness skin graft.

Grafting the sinus walls stops formation of polypoid tissue and mucus generation within the sinus and allows the walls to become load-bearing areas .[23]

With the increased use of osseointegrated implants, dependence on mechanical and anatomic methods of retention has diminished. Osseointegrated implants provide excellent retention to the definitive obturator.

Retentive magnets and various designs of clips are available to minimize force transfer to the implant and supporting bone .[22]

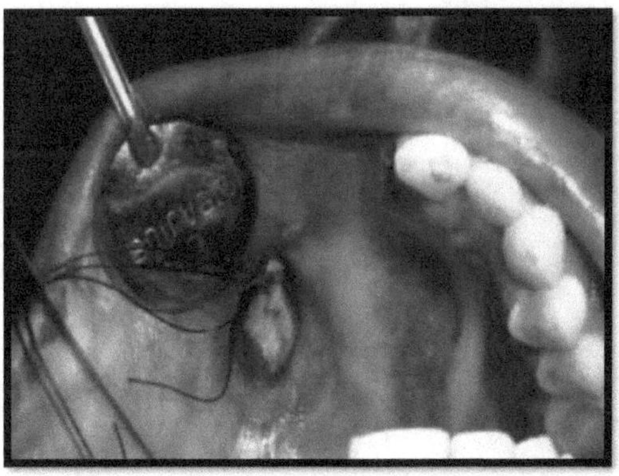

Healed maxillary defect

FIGURE:29

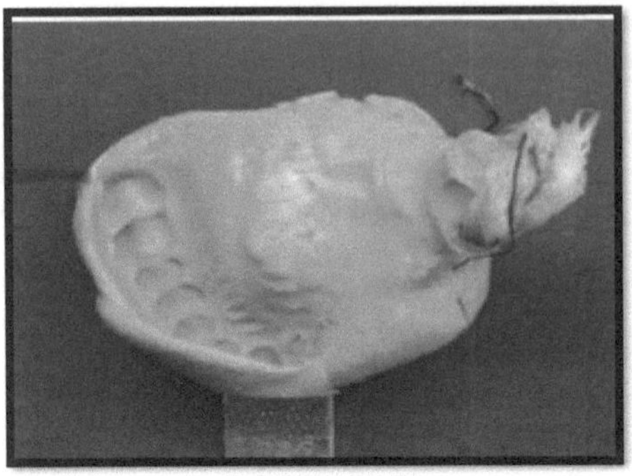

Impression made in irreversible hydrocolloid

FIGURE:30

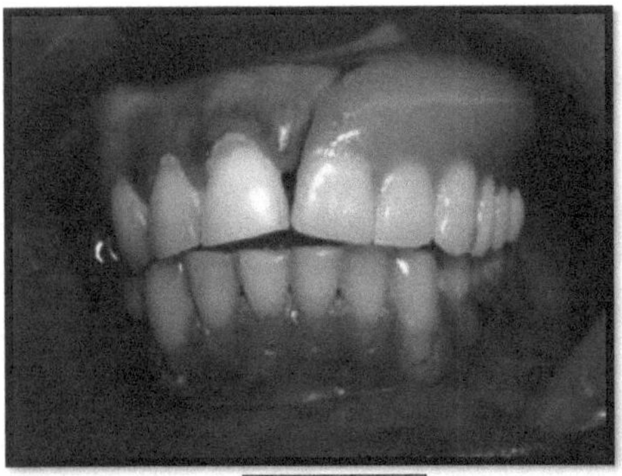

Try in of maxillary obturator prosthesis

FIGURE:31

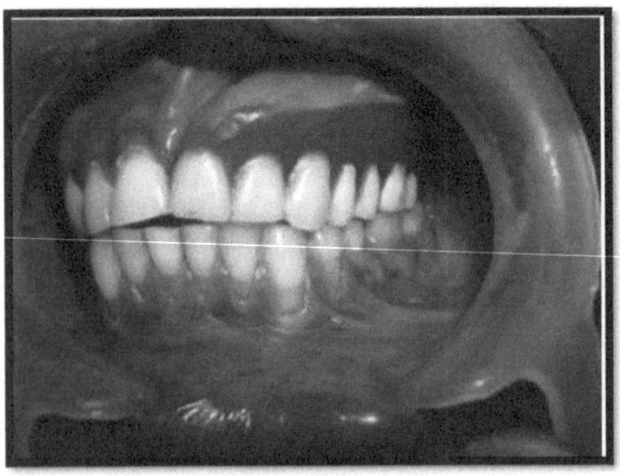

Interim obturator prosthesis in situ

FIGURE:32

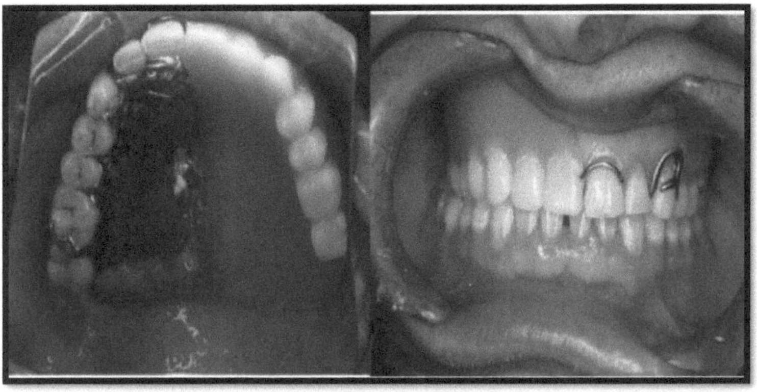

FIGURE:33

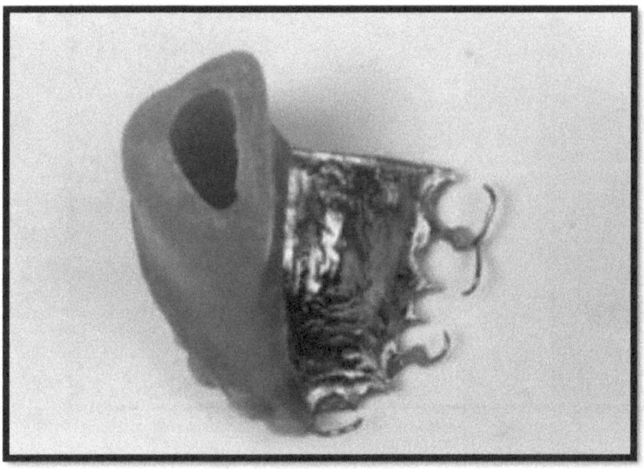

FIGURE:34

Definitive obturator prosthesis FIGURE:33

Definitive obturator prosthesis showing hollow bulb FIGURE:34

EXTRA ORAL IMPLANTS

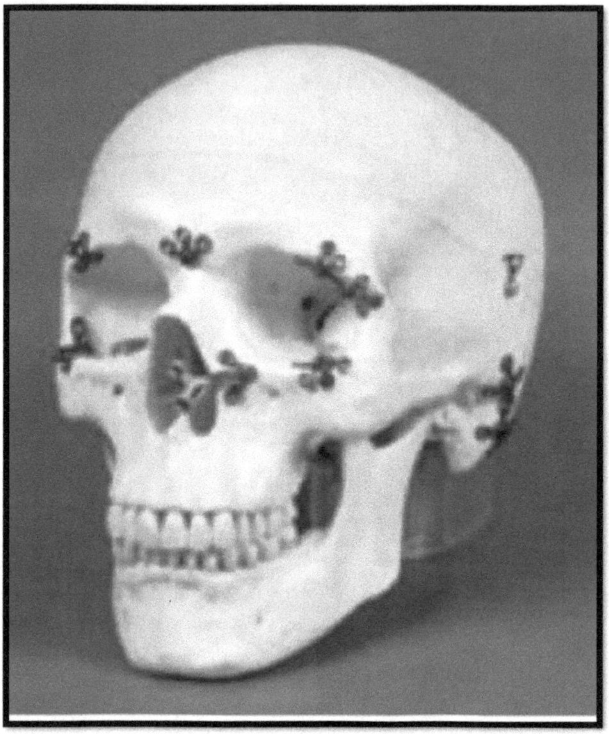

FIGURE:35

1. **ORBITAL (OCULAR) IMPLANTS**

It is used to replace enucleated eyes. One should remember that the lacrimal apparatus (eyelids and associated glands) is intact. In these patients the prosthesis only replaces the eyeball.

- The impression is made with irreversible hydrocolloids. For the reduction of mucosal sensitivity the orbit is treated by anesthetics. Colloid must be in liquid condition.
- A special tray is fabricated.
- The secondary impression is made with the second layer of irreversible hydrocolloids.
- Casts are poured in two sections with two keyways in the first pour and separating medium.
- Sclera is fabricated with wax.
- It is tried in the eye socket and evaluated for lid contours.
- Following which, it is flasked and de-waxed.
- Special sclera white acrylic resin is available for such procedures. • Scleral resin is packed, processed, trimmed and polished as usual. • Next the ocular ball prosthesis is tried in the patient's defect.
- The position of the iris is determined during the trial procedure. The patient is made to relax. The dentist should mark the location of the iris by comparing it with the unaffected eye on the other side.
- The iris is placed and fused to the sclera prosthesis. A cut back is created in the sclera to seat the iris button.
- Characteristic pigmentations on the iris can be applied according to the shade of the other eye.[24]

  This procedure is known as Iris painting.

It is done in three parts or phases namely:

1. The pupil
2. Base colour
3. Detailed colorate.

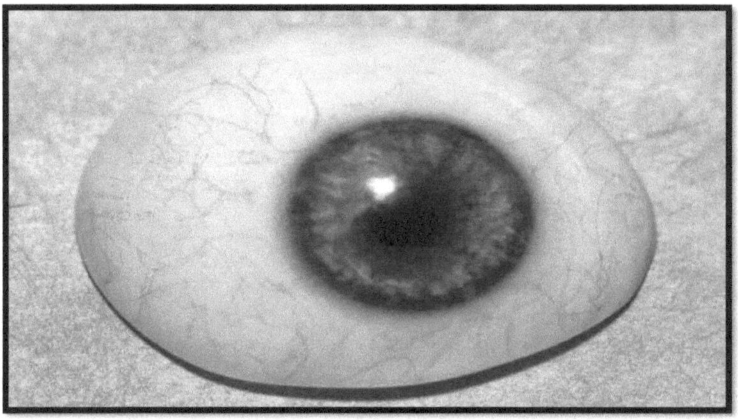

FIGURE:36

Osseointegrated implants are an extraoral alternative for the rehabilitation of patients suffering from facial mutilation due to trauma, cancer or congenital diseases. According to J. Wolfaardt, the main benefits of implant-supported oral-maxillofacial prosthesis treatments over reconstructive surgery are:

- Surgery is shorter.
- Surgical risk is lower.
- The procedure can be performed under local anesthesia.
- The results are more predictable than with autogenous grafts.

- There is no donor site.
- There is lower morbidity .
- It is possible to monitor the tumor resection site to diagnose and provide early treatment in case of potential relapse.

Contraindications:

- Psychiatric illnesses and untreated addictive behaviors.
- Failure to keep implants in proper hygienic conditions (which jeopardizes the prognosis) .
- When the patient is not easily accessible in order to sustain a proper maintenance therapy.[25]

The treatment options for patients who need oculo-palpebral prosthesis are:

- Eye patch: This treatment is not aesthetically pleasing, nor does it offer proper .protection against cold temperatures.
- Surgical reconstruction: it has high morbidity, it is not aesthetically pleasing and it blocks tumor relapse monitoring in cancer patients. In addition, there is no surgical procedure to rehabilitate the eyeball .
- Prostheses retained by adhesive, mechanical or anatomical means:

  - Mechanical: Eyeglass frames and acrylic pieces are the most commonly used retention devices for facial prostheses.

  Eyeglass frames are excellent for nasal and oculo-palpebral prostheses retention. However, many patients become distressed when they have to remove the prosthesis together with the frame.

- Anatomical: These may be used as retainers in anatomical cavities through soft material extensions or acrylic structures, when the support tissues around the cavity are healthy.

- Adhesives: Skin adhesives may cause contact allergies, lose adhesion with perspiration and have poor effectiveness, depending on the prosthesis size and weight. In addition, some patients report difficulties when refitting the prostheses.

- Prosthesis on implants:

It is the treatment of choice for defects of this nature. The use of implants has reduced the number of problems associated to the integrity of the prosthesis edges, the difficulties patients experience when repositioning them and they also make it possible to camouflage their borders.

Advantages of prostheses over implants are:

- excellent retention
- simple connection for the patient
- no skin damage
- longer lifespan
- better aesthetic results.

Pre-surgical prosthetic planning :

1. **Pre-surgical information:**

It is important to collect as much information as possible about the patient's physical features before the surgical procedure. This can be done by observing pictures, using models, profiling instruments, etc.

2. **Pre-surgical and pre-prosthetic psychological assessment.**

It is essential to evaluate the patient's expectations and to determine the suitability of the treatment .

3. **Model analysis.**

Before placing the implants it is essential to develop models for diagnostic study and to make the surgical guides .

These can be made out of resin or vinyl-acetate based on the wax sculptures.

Some guides can be obtained by 3D modeling and attached to bone tissue.

The less invasive ones can be attached to the teeth in the upper jaw.

4. **Sculpture:**

Before making the sculpture it is necessary to define the extension, which should be as limited as possible, so the prosthesis is unnoticeable.

Then, a wax film is tailored to the model and the operator may use wax for the entire sculpture or modeling clay, as recommended by the Sao Paulo Brazilian school.

This is a replication stage, where we must consider facial proportions and apply our knowledge of artistic anatomy, physical anthropology and facial mapping. It is important to consider every detail on the healthy side, or whatever source of information selected, whether it be pictures of the patient, relatives, etc.

5. **Imaging studies:**

To place extraoral implants it is essential to have a CT scan. The scan makes it possible to produce a prototype, through a modeling process (stereolithography) that integrates different technologies.

This enables us to obtain a three-dimensional materialization of the structures identified in the CT scan in a life-size 1:1 scale, which is very useful to map the surgery.[24]

Surgical technique

General surgical considerations:

According to Badie, the three main sites to place extraoral implants are:

- The temporal region
- The oculo-palpebral region
- The naso-maxillary region.

The supraorbital margin is typically used in the oculo-palpebral region, as it is possible to place 3-4 mm-long implants, or even longer ones sometimes, depending on the assessment previously made based on the X-rays or CT scans.

The success rate for the oculo-palpebral region is lower than for the temporal region, as the margin is thin and there is low bone density.

Wolfaardt recommends using implants with no expanded platform in this area, since the risk of exposure is high as the bone is thin.

He advises surgeons to be particularly careful not to affect the appearance of the eyebrow when repositioning the flap. Based on this, dental implants is the option selected in this clinical case as their design is more suitable for the orbital region.

Nowadays, there are tapered implants available with a smaller diameter and more robust threads to compensate low bone density.

This makes it possible to achieve good primary stability .

It is essential to apply the right surgical technique to achieve good prosthetic results and to preserve the health of the peri-implant tissue.

Soft tissue needs to be handled effectively.

In preparation, hair follicles need to be removed from the area surrounding the implants.

Subcutaneous tissue must be removed in approximately 10 mm around the implant area .

Therefore, the ideal peri-implant tissue will be thin, motionless, with no hair follicles and no ridges.

Potential implant sites in this region are:

- the upper
- lateral and
- lower orbital ridge

where it is possible to place 3-4 mm-long implants, as previously stated. About three to four implants are necessary to retain these prostheses.

The longitudinal axis of the implant should be positioned towards the center of the orbit.

The surgical guide will be essential to identify the position of the implants, so these do not interfere with that of the ocular prosthesis. Transepithelial pillars must be kept within the limits of the orbital cavity so as not to affect the prosthesis.

The use of surgical guides is fundamental and so is the presence of the rehabilitation professionals during the procedure.[25]

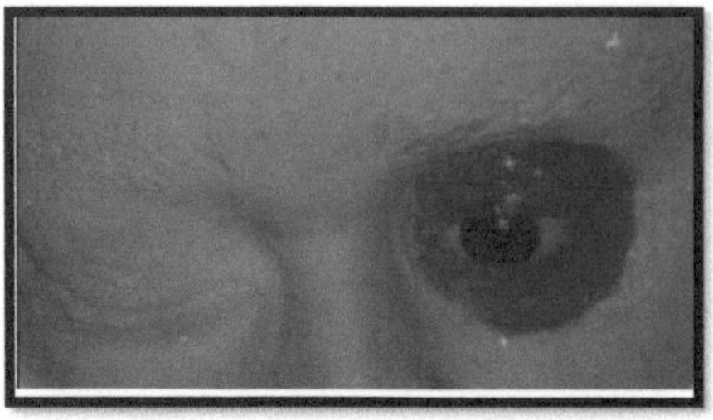

Diagnostic study model with wax diagnostic sculpture

FIGURE:37

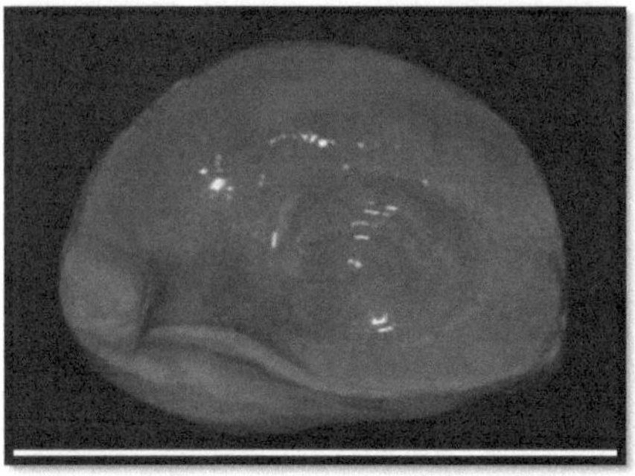

Diagnostic model duplicate and stamped surgical guide

FIGURE:38

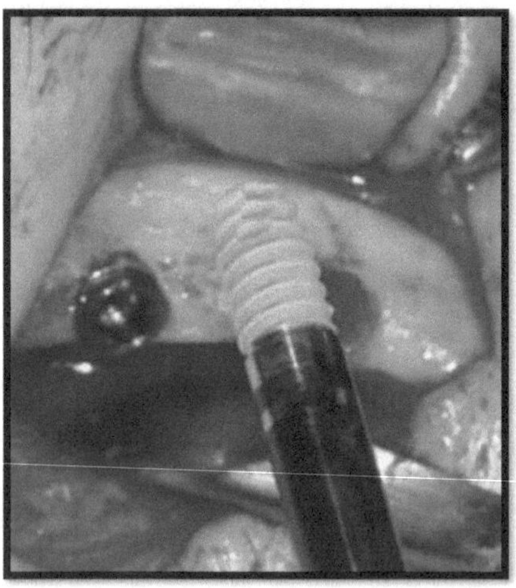

Tapered implants, short (8.5 mm) and reduced diameter (3.25 mm)

FIGURE:39

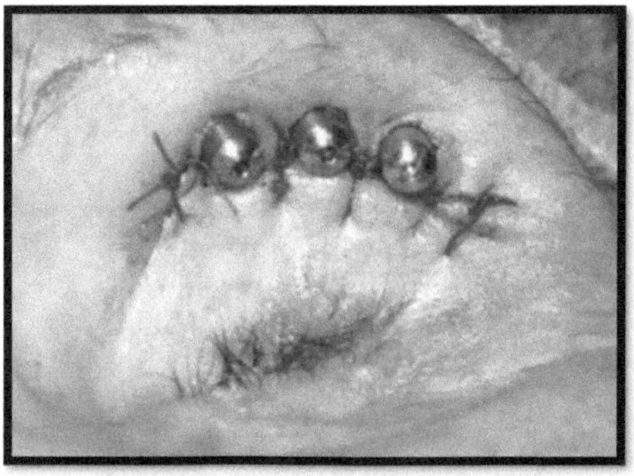

Soft tissue suture with 4.0 nylon suture

FIGURE:40

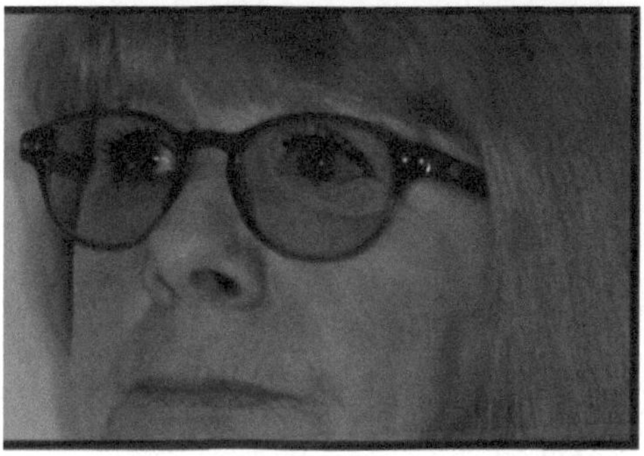

Prosthesis in place

FIGURE:41

Using dental implants for rehabilitation with oral-maxillofacial prostheses is a suitable treatment option.[26]

2)

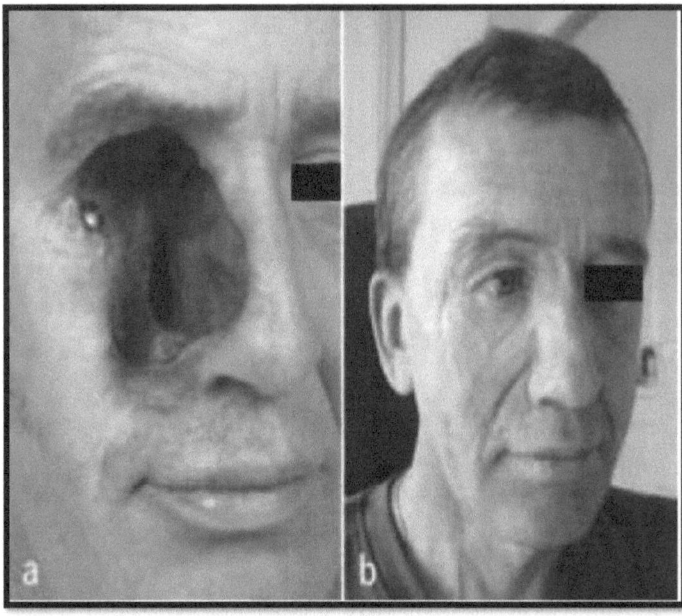

FIGURE:42 a) In patient implants have been exposed and temporarily covered with healing caps until the magnets are screwed on. From this angle the cranial implant is not visible. The split thickness skin graft placed into the cavity has healed in. b)The patient is wearing the bone –anchored facial prosthesis(Epitheseninstitut Schneider)

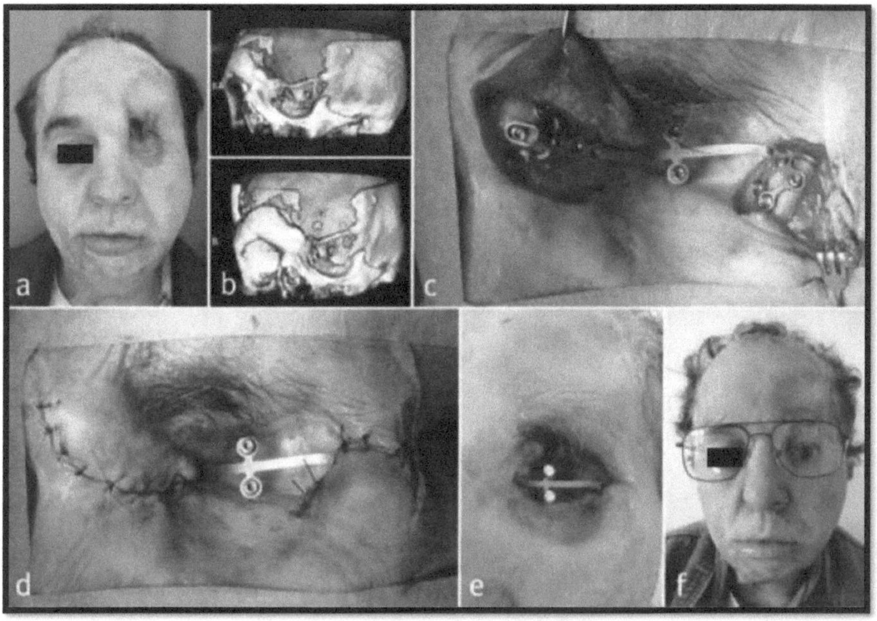

FIGURE:43 a) 49 year-old patient with a fronto-orbital facial defect 3 years after craniofacial resection. b) The bone defect is recognisable in the CT. The most important anchorage option in the region of the cranial orbital clip is missing. c) The long plate of the Epiplating system is fixed subperiostally in the region of the glabella and to the malar bone. The thread guides are secured by covering screws and lie in the centre of the orbital cavity. d) The wound is closed. e) The healing process is complete. Magnets (Steco) are screwed into the thread guides. f) The patient is provided with a bone-anchored orbital prosthesis (Epitheseninstitut Schneider). The patient wears glasses for improved camouflage and protection of the right eye.[27]

2. NASAL PROSTHESIS

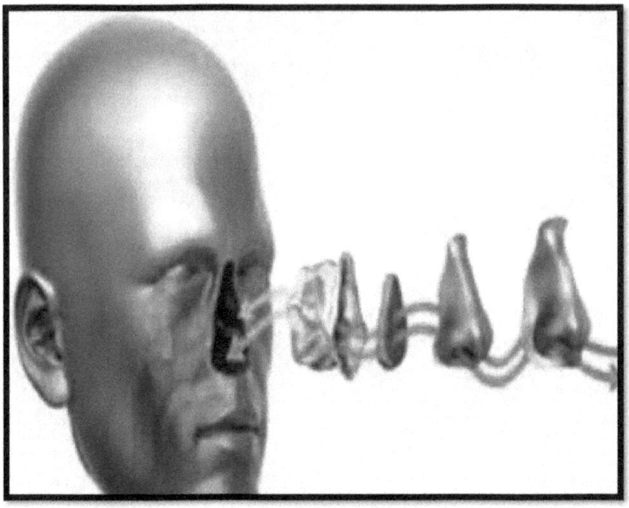

FIGURE:44

Patients with maxillofacial defects have been challenging to treat. A multitude of challenges associated with maxillofacial prosthetic treatment are not typically seen with patients who need conventional prosthodontic treatment. These types of patients generally require replacement of significant amounts of hard and soft tissues than do conventional prosthodontic patient.[28]

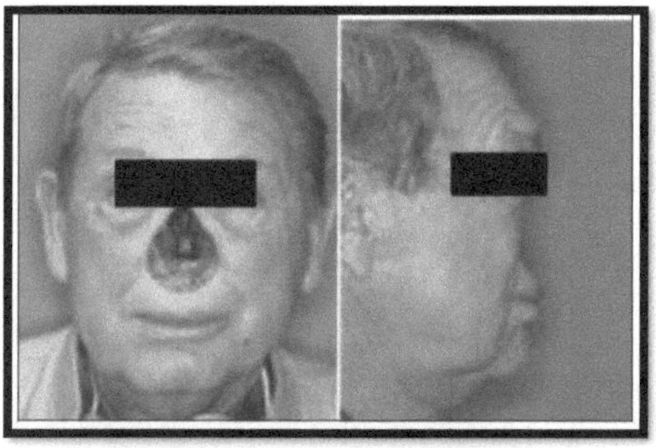

Preoperative frontal and lateral views of the patient.

FIGURE:45

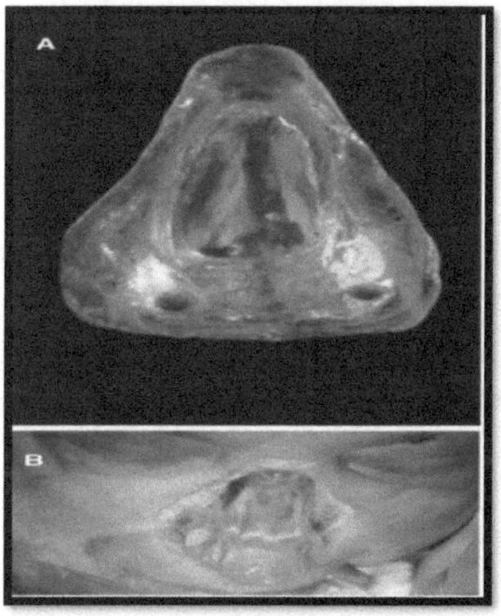

Clear acrylic resin stent (A) and a coronal view of the patient with the acrylic resin stent in place (B).

FIGURE:46

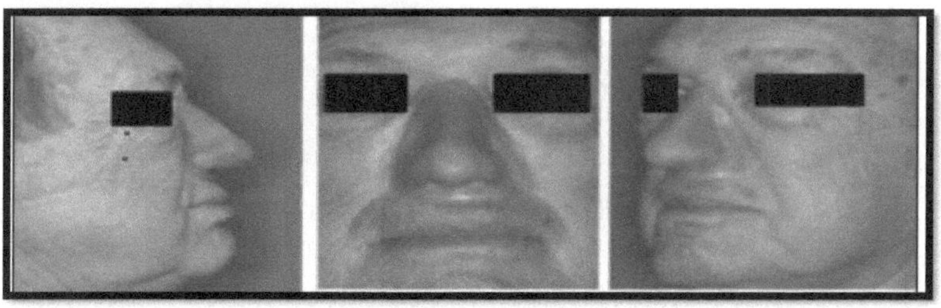

3 Lateral, frontal, and left three-fourth views of the patient with the wax prosthesis.

FIGURE:47

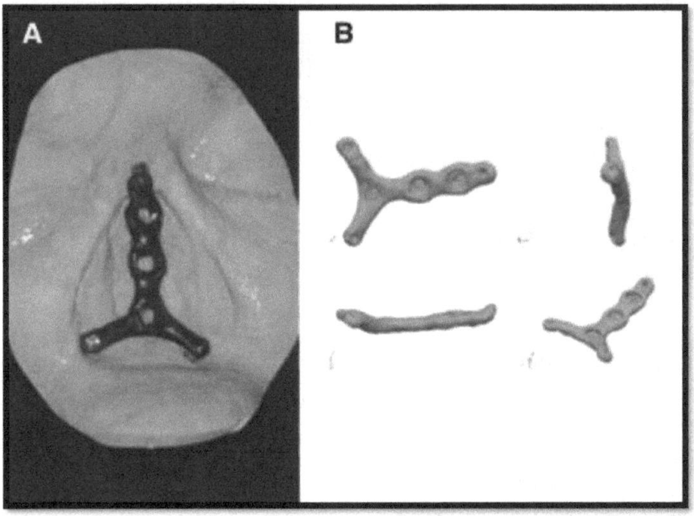

FIGURE:48

CAD/CAM framework (A) Framework in place in the extraoral cast (B) Various views of the CAD/CAM images of the wax pattern/framework.

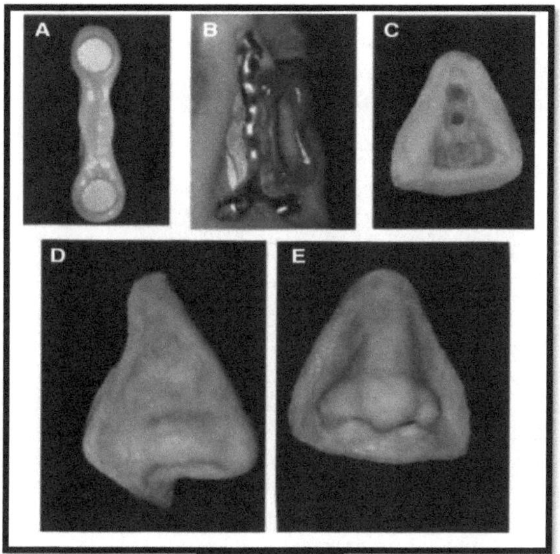

FIGURE:49

(A, B) Magnetic housings for prosthesis (C) Posterior view of the silicone prosthesis. Lateral (D) and frontal (E) views of the finished silicone prosthesis.

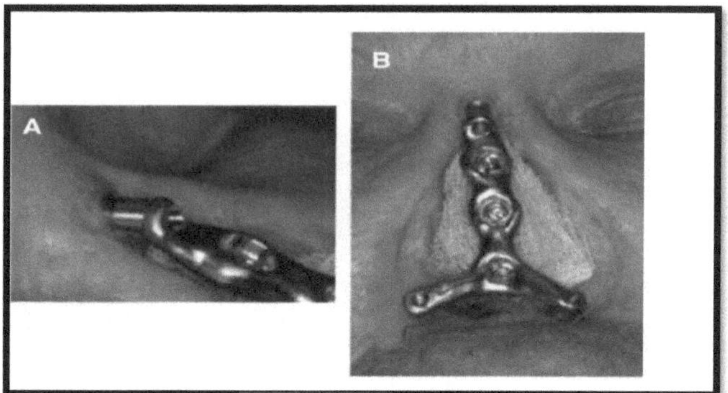

FIGURE:50

The framework in place on the patient (A) Close-up view of the superior abutment screw in the framework (B) Frontal view of the framework on the patient

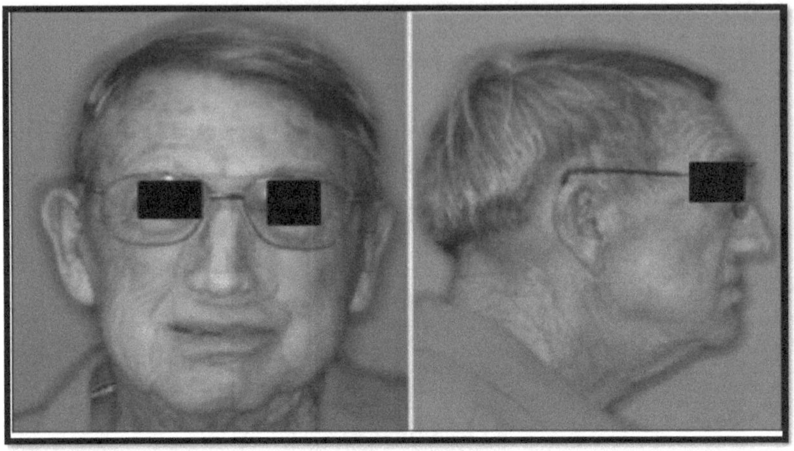

FIGURE:51

Frontal and lateral views of the patient with the completed nasal prosthesis in place.[28]

#2 Due to the limited amount of bone available, the use of solitary implants in the nasal region is problematic.

Provided that the nasal bone is completely removed, sufficient bone can be found around the glabella.

Anchoring a nasal prosthesis to a solitary Brånemark implant in the glabella is possible.

Otherwise solitary implants can be used solely at the nasal floor which, however, provides less a secure retention for the prosthesis.

Good bone availability for the use of the Epiplating system can be found around the piriform aperture, and in particular at the frontal process of the maxilla .[29]

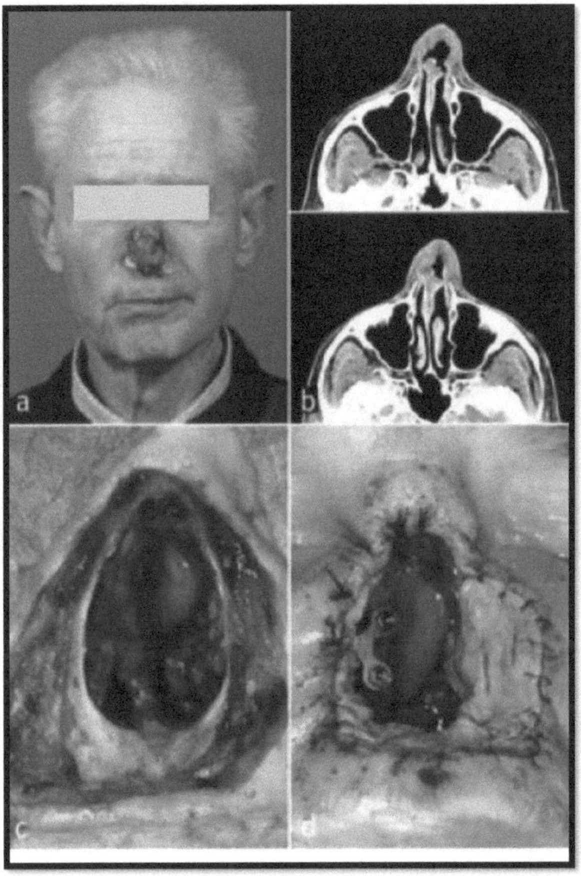

FIGURE:52

a) 67 year-old patient with a squamous cell carcinoma of the inner nose. Recurrence after primary radiotherapy 1 year earlier. b) The CT shows widespread infiltration. c) Intra-operative situation following tumour resection. d) An Epiplating nasal plate is inserted on the right. The tapped holes are secured with blue covering screws. Open wound areas are covered with split thickness skin transplants.

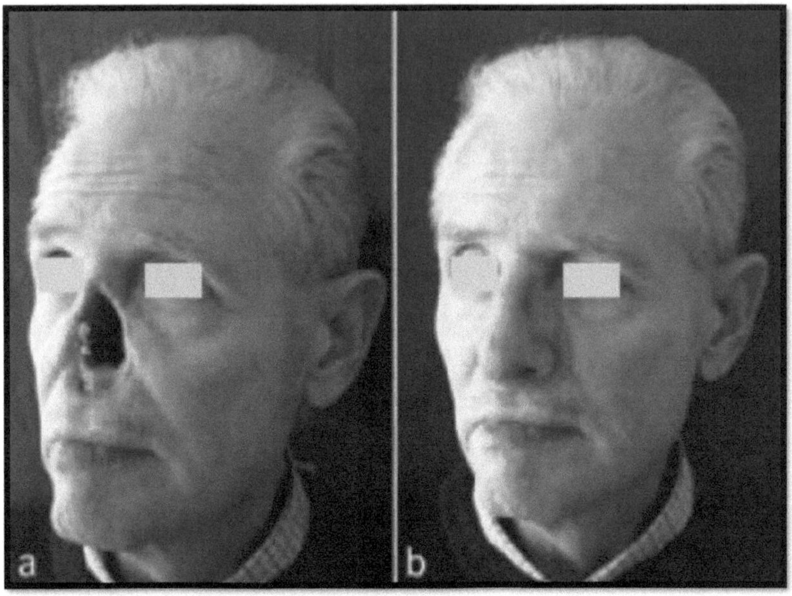

FIGURE:53

a) Patient two months after surgery. The implant is stable with no adverse skin reactions and is fitted with 2 magnet inserts (Steco). b) Patient with the bone-anchored nasal prosthesis (Epitheseninstitut Schneider)[29]

AURICULAR PROSTHESIS

The auricle may be congenitally malformed as in microtia or may be disfigured as a result of trauma following road traffic accidents, burns, acid attacks, or animal or human bites.

Surgically they may be removed due to local malignancies.

Plastic surgeons may attempt an autogenous reconstruction of the external ear but it is extremely challenging and technically demanding.

In contrast an esthetically pleasing and excellent shade matched auricular prosthesis may be fabricated from acrylic polymers or from silicone elastomers.

The main problem with these prostheses has been their retention. Traditionally tissue undercuts, mechanical retention with springs, clips, hairpieces and adhesives have been used to hold them in place. These have serious limitations as retention is not very strong and can be dislodged by daily activities of life .[8]

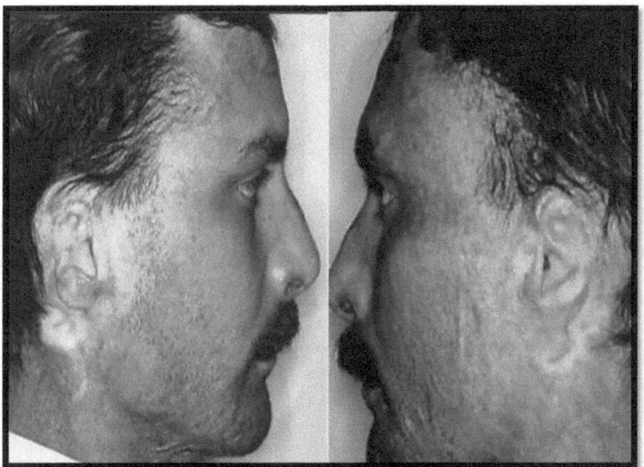

FIGURE:54

Bilateral auricular defect following severe burns

In this case, two or three implants placed external to the external auditory meatus in the temporo-mastoid region are sufficient . Implants placed to retain a prosthetic ear are limited in length by the thickness of the mastoid and temporal bones as well as the mastoid air cells.

Positioning of implants in the temporal bone is critical to the overall esthetic result and so the use of a surgical guide is mandatory.

In cases of microtia or where there are a malformed tissue tags it may be beneficial to have them surgically removed prior to the start of the rehabilitation process .[30]

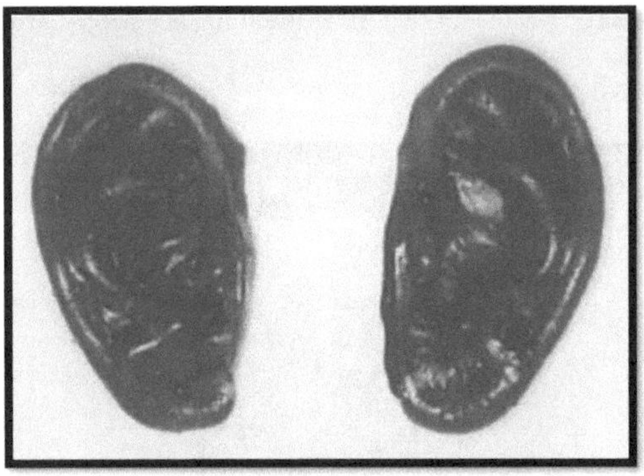

Wax pattern of ear prosthesis

FIGURE:55

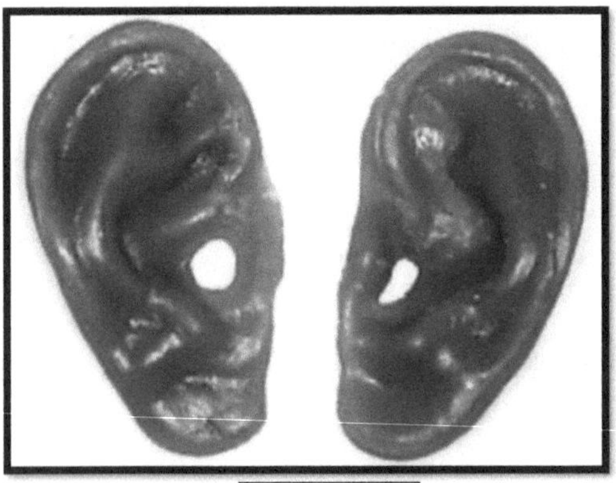

Finished and polished silicone ear prosthesis

FIGURE:56

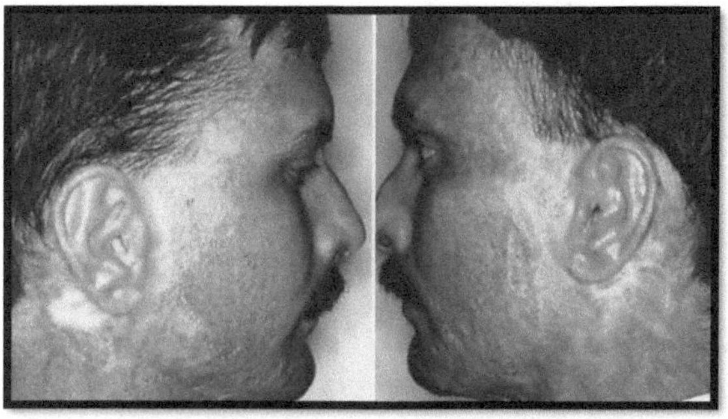

FIGURE:57

Bilateral auricular prosthesis (mechanically retained)

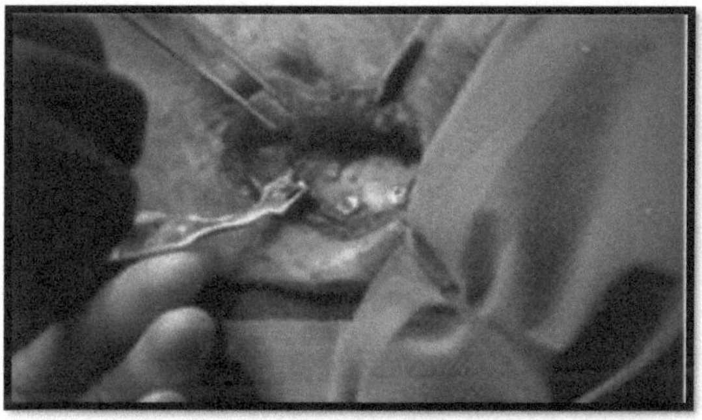

FIGURE:58

Craniofacial implants placed for ear prosthesis

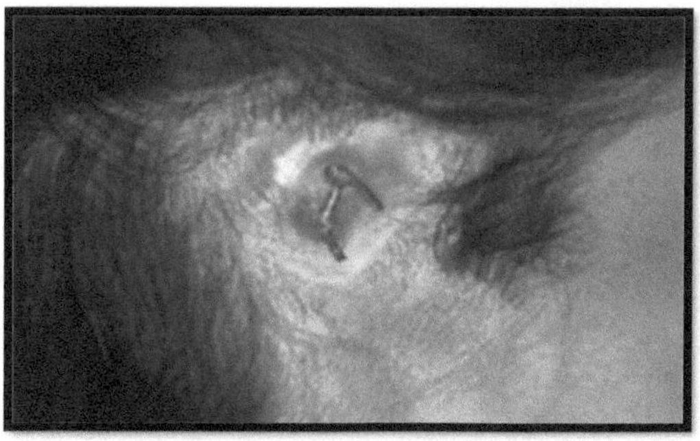

FIGURE:59

Bar retainer connected to abutment

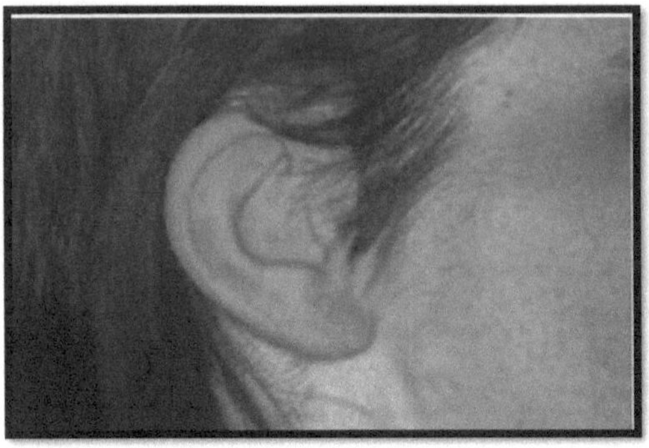

FIGURE:60

Implant retained ear prosthesis in situ

2) A 22-year-old male with left congenital ear loss was referred to the Dental and Maxillofacial Prosthetic Department of Dental School of Isfahan University of Medical Sciences.

First of all, a surgical stent should be made.

The impression was made with irreversible hydrocolloid from both ears.

Hence, a wax-up for left ear was made to predict proper position of implants to achieve natural future prosthesis and according to the right ear position and form. The wax-up was flasked to make surgical stent. Computed tomography evaluation of mastoid bone was done in coronal, sagittal, and axial planes.

The implants were placed by one-stage surgery.

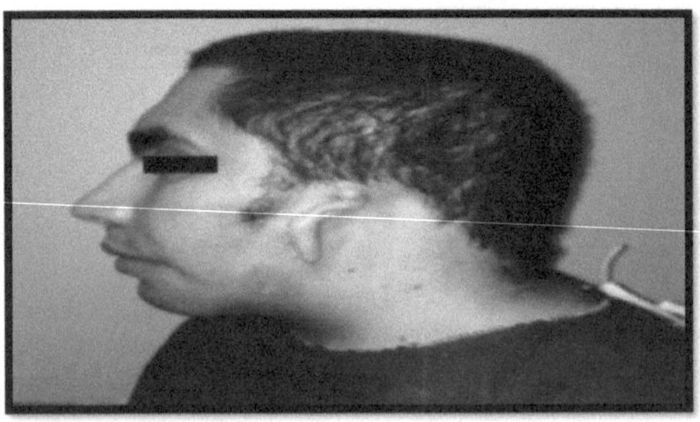

FIGURE:61

Primary view

Two 6 mm length and 4.2 mm width dental implants (SIC max screw implant, Birmannsgasse, Switzerland) were placed in the mastoid bone, and the thickness of soft tissue was reduced .

For prosthetic procedure, use of Safe On Four system was done because bar and bridge abutment could be used as a transcutaneous component and was fixed with a screw separately from second part of abutment. Immediately after placement of fixtures, bar and bridge abutment of Safe On four system (SIC Fixation Postsafe on Four, GH 3.0 mm Birmannsgasse, Switzerland) was closed to the fixtures and proper healing screw (SIC Gingiva Shaper Safe on Four, cylindrical) was closed.

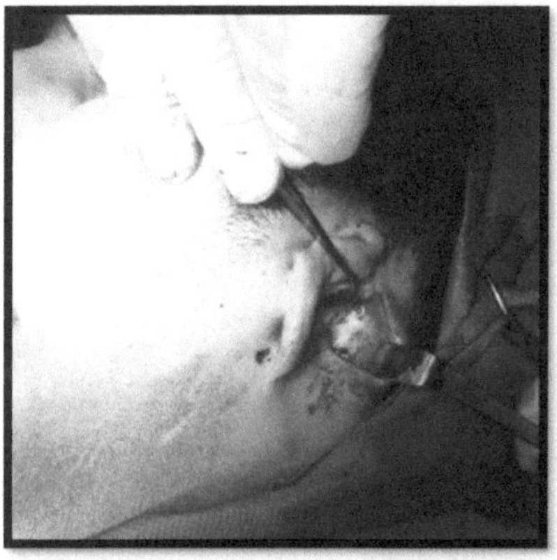

FIGURE:62

Implants placement

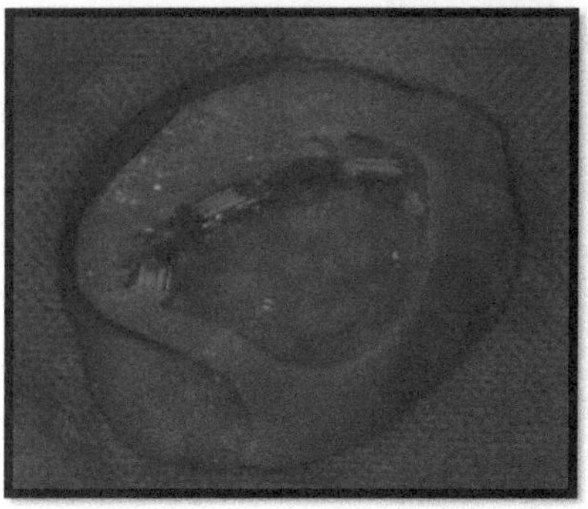

FIGURE:63

Final prostheses skin surface

After 3 months impression coping were closed to the abutments and the impression was made at abutment level.

The cast was prepared and UCLA abutments were closed to the first abutment analogs. Then, a round plastic bar was attached to UCLA abutments.

The bar was prepared for casting. After preparation of bar, proper housings and clips were selected.

Acrylic resin was placed on housings and bar to make substructure for silicon. A thin layer of wax was formed under acrylic substructure to provide dry environment around skin surface of abutment.

A wax-up was made on this substructure. Then, the wax-up was tried on the face and was accepted by the patient. The waxed model was flasked. The primer was rubbed to the acrylic substructure to gain proper bond to silicone.

The silicone which was colored with intrinsic pigments, and flakes, similar to the right normal ear was entered to the flask. After setting completed, extrinsic pigments (Cosmesil Dry Pigment, PRINCIPALITY, Newport, Wales, UK) were used to mimic surrounding tissues colors.[31]

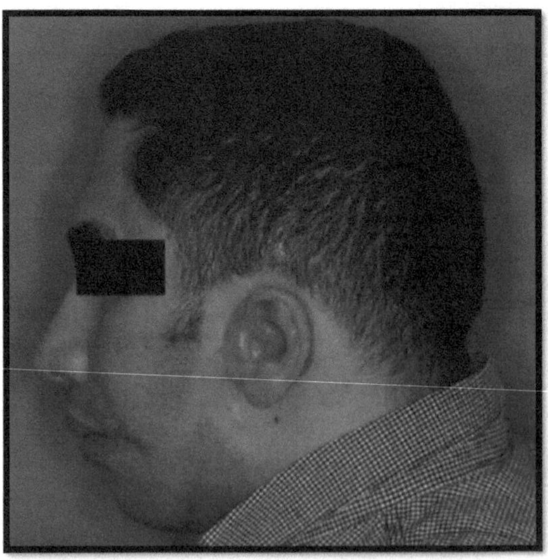

FIGURE:64

Final view

3 CASE STUDY:

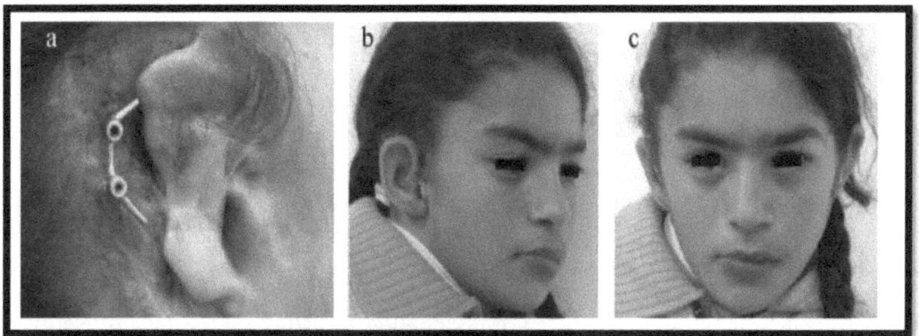

FIGURE:65

(a) Close up of the defect area in patient , showing soldered Dolder bars and bar abutments screwed in implant abutments; (b) lateral and (c) frontal view of the patient with auricular prosthesis in place.[31]

BAHA

Bone-anchored hearing aids (BAHA) are indicated in patients with conductive or mixed hearing loss unsuitable for conventional air conduction hearing aids and ineligible for surgical rehabilitation.[32]

These hearing aids, initially developed by Tjellström and Carlsson (Göteborg) in 1977, are based on the concept of osseointegration described by Branemark.

Due to the presence of a foreign body in contact with the scalp, skin reactions are commonly observed and can sometimes lead to severe complications:

- Skin necrosis
- Infection
- Hypertrophic scar
- Defective osseointegration possibly responsible for fixture loss.

The BAHA surgical implantation procedure is simple, but requires compliance with certain basic principles to minimize the postoperative complication rate.[33]

Many surgical variants concerning the skin incision have been described, all designed to reduce these complications. Few techniques are mentioned below.

ANTERIOR BASED SKIN FLAP TECHNIQUE:

In the skin flap technique, a 3 to 4 cm rectangular or semicircular incision centered on the implant position is performed .

The scalpel is not placed perpendicular to cortical bone, but at an angle in order to harvest a maximum of subcutaneous tissue present underneath the edges of the skin around the implant.

The flap is then reclined anteriorly, sparing the periosteum which must be simply perforated over the site of implantation of the screw.

The fixture is then inserted according to the principles described by Branemark: a countersink, 3 or 4 mm long depending on the thickness of the bone, is drilled using a high speed cutting drill.

This countersink is then enlarged with a bone rasp to the shape and diameter of the implant.

Finally, a 3 or 4 mm self-tapping fixture is screwed at low speed perpendicularly to the bone.

All these procedures must be performed under abundant irrigation to prevent heating of the bone that can interfere with osseointegration.

The skin flap is subsequently thinned with a scalpel blade, in a subdermal plane removing the hair follicles: the flap must be hairless to facilitate subsequent cleaning, and must be as thin as possible. Removal of part of the subcutaneous tissue of the peri-implant skin achieves a gently sloping junction with the implantation site.

Finally, the flap is placed over the fixture, sutured with 5.0 monofilament, and perforated over the fixture with a punch scalpel, and the abutment is then screwed onto the fixture.

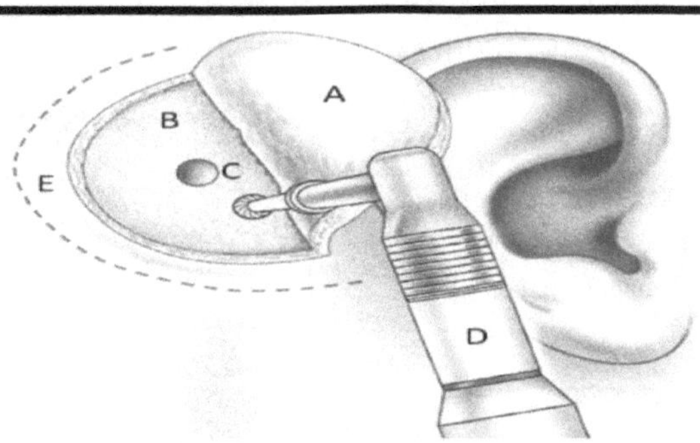

Anterior-based skin flap technique. A. Anterior-based flap. B. Periosteum. C. Countersink. D. 2 or 3 mm long cutting drill. E. Zone of thinning of the subcutaneous tissue around the implant.

FIGURE:66

SKIN GRAFT TECHNIQUE:

The skin graft technique is similar to the skin flap technique except that the incision is circular (3 to 4 cm in diameter) .

Implantation of the fixture and abutmentis performed according to the same principles. The skin graft is thinned in the same way as the flap, with removal of all hair follicles.

At the end of operation, a healing cap is clipped onto the abutment, underneath which a piece of tulle gras is placed to act as a compressive dressing.

This cap and the sutures are removed on the 10th postoperative day. The processor is installed 6 to 8 weeks after the operation.

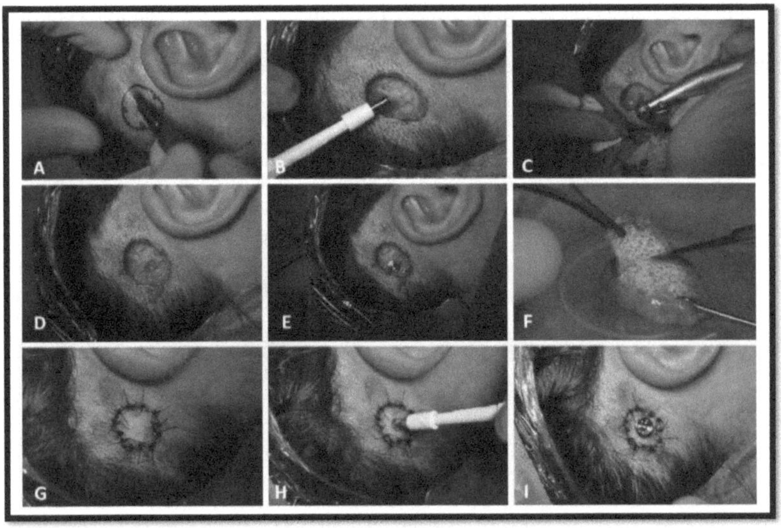

FIGURE:67

Circular full-thickness skin graft technique. A. Oblique circular incision. B. Creation of a periosteal window using the punch scalpel. C. High-speed drilling of the countersink. D. Reaming of the countersink. E. Placement of the fixture. F. Subdermal thinning of the graft. G. Suture of the graft. H. Perforation in the centre of the graft. I. Placement of the abutment.

Complications were classified into four categories:

- Flap/graft necrosis;

- Inflammation/infection;
- Hypertrophic scar;
- Primary or secondary defective osseointegration of the fixture.

BAHA implants have been demonstrated to be effective in some patients with conductive hearing loss and, to a lesser extent, unilateral cophosis.

BAHAs can be implanted according to several techniques, mainly dermatome, skin flap, skin graft or a single vertical incision.

Skin complications, especially hypertrophic scar around the abutment, are frequent and represent the main disadvantage of these implants.

Very variable results concerning complications have been reported in the literature and no technique has been clearly demonstrated to be superior. [34]

PROSTHETIC REHABILITATION IN PARRY ROMBERG SYNDROME PATIENT.

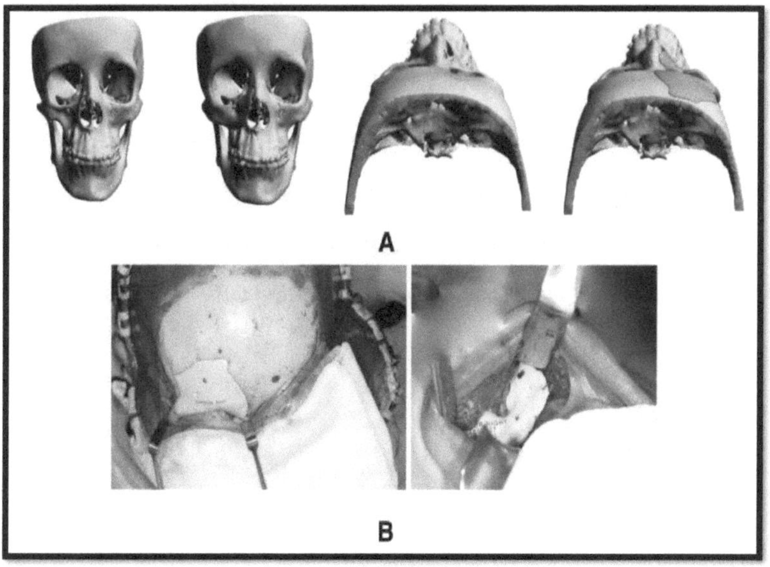

FIGURE:68

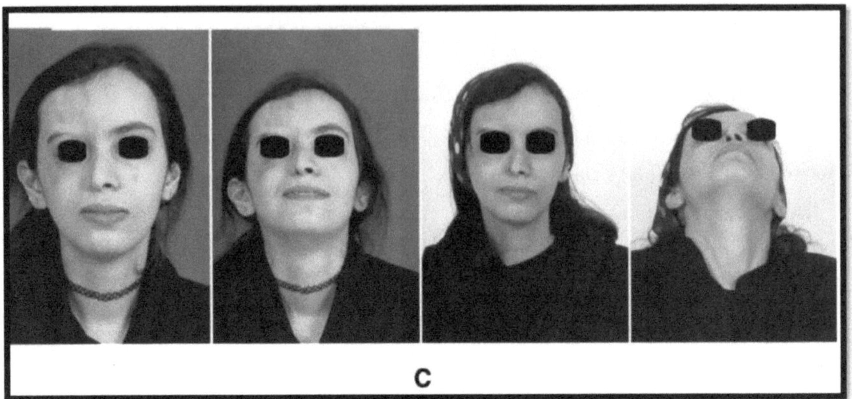

FIGURE:69

Parry-Romberg syndrome case. a 3D reconstruction of the CT showing the defects and the planned implants. b Intraoperative views of the implants. c Pre- and postoperative photographs of the patient.

Case 1: A 23-year-old female was diagnosed with Parry-romberg syndrome, resulting in hypoplasia in the right side of her face. Patient had a history of fat grafting and fillers to cover the defect with unsatisfactory results. The patient underwent PEEK PSI reconstruction for her frontal bone, zygoma, and maxilla on the right side of her face through bicoronal and vestibular approaches. Patient satisfaction was reported as excellent postoperatively.[35]

MATERIALS USED AS IMPLANTS IN MAXILLOFACIAL PROSTHESIS

The history of masking maxillofacial defects dates centuries back when the Egyptians and Chinese used wax and resins to reconstruct missing portion of the head and neck region .

This journey of searching an ideal material was started since 1500 A.D (when facial prostheses were described by French surgeon Ambrose Pare in 1575) and have evolved from earlier prosthesis, made from gold, silver, paper, cloth, leather, wrought, metals, ceramics, vulcanite, acrylic to latex, polyvinyl chloride and copolymers, chlorinated polyethylene, polyurethane elastomers, medical grade silicones and polyposphazines.

Silicones, were introduced in 1946, but were used for the first time by Barnhart (1960) for extra-oral prosthesis and became more popular over other materials .[36]

Acrylic resins –

Particularly used in cases where there is least movement of tissue bed during function.

Advantages :

- Its ready availability
- Colour stability
- Can be relined and repaired
- Have good strength
- Can be fabricated with feather margin
- Good shelf life of about two years.

However, they are rigid, have water absorption and duplication is not possible.

Disadvantages:

- poor edge strength
- poor durability
- degradation when exposed to sunlight.

The restoration often becomes tacky and predisposes to dust collection and staining.

New generation of acrylic monomers, oligomers and macromeres are thermal, chemical and photo initiated and can eliminate the short comings of traditional acrylic co-polymers .

Polyvinylchloride and copolymer-

A clear, tasteless and odorless material and has been used widely for maxillo-facial applications with advantages like being flexible, adaptable to both intrinsic and extrinsic staining.

Plasticizers are added to produce an elastomeric effect at room temperature.

Other ingredients include cross-linking agents for added strength and ultraviolet stabilizers for colour stability.[37]

Chlorinated polyethylene-

Processing involves high heat curing pigmented sheets in metal molds.

Dow chemicals' chlorinated polyethylene elastomer is an industrial grade thermoplastic elastomer.

It is less irritating to the mucosa than silicone, less toxic than thermosetting silicone materials and non carcinogenic.

Chlorinated polyethylene elastomer appears to be a suitable substitute for silicones for the fabrication of extraoral maxillofacial prosthesis in situations where cost of silicone is prohibitive.[36]

Polyurethane elastomers

- This material is chemically composed of an extended segment of aliphatic diisocyanate groups and a segment of polyol groups (a mixture of polyesters) and an organotin catalyst for the polymerization process to occur.

Advantages:

- Stability
- Higher tear resistance
- Low modulus without use of plasticizers
- Good ultimate strength and
- Elongation.

They can accept intrinsic colouration and are amenable to maxillofacial processing technique.

Disadvantages :

- poor colour stability
- poor compatibility with adhesive systems
- moisture sensitivity leading to gas bubbles during processing, this due to presence of diisocynates which also account for the toxicity of the material.
  Reaction must be carried out in dry atmosphere or carbon dioxide will be produced and porous elastomer results .

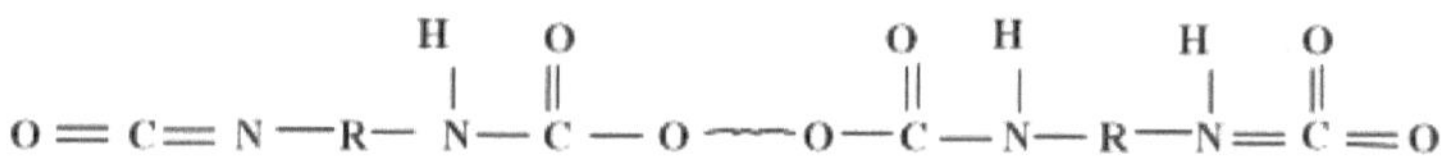

Polyurethane

Thermoset urethane elastomers

are produced through introduction of primary chemical crosslinks. If reactants are combined in Stoichiometric ratios and reactions are preferentially catalysed, a known controlled morphology can be developed. In one study polyurethane was greatly affected by aging .

Silicones

Also known as **polydimethyl siloxane** is the most successful maxillofacial prosthetic material till now and the new advances are being made to this material to overcome their weaknesses.

- These became more popular over other materials as they have a range of good physical properties (such as excellent tear and tensile strength)
- Over a range of temperature
- Easier to manipulate
- High degree of chemical inertness

- Low degree of toxicity
- High degree of thermal and oxidative stability.

Further they can be stained intrinsically and/or extrinsically to give them more lifelike natural appearance.

When adequately cured, silicones elastomers resist absorbing organic materials that lead to bacterial growth and so with simple cleaning these materials are relatively safe and sanitary compared to other materials .

Silicone is a combination of organic and inorganic compounds and chemically they are termed as polydimethyl siloxane.

The inorganic backbone makes the unique difference of this material as siloxane bonds Si—O—Si in the main chains, as well as Si—C bonds where side groups are bonded to silicone, are extremely flexible and have a great freedom of motion.

This is reflected in their lower viscosity, lower surface tension, lower melting point and glass transition temperatures, and is responsible for the elastomeric behaviors of many polysiloxanes. Polyurethane Polydimethyl Siloxane As these segments are varied in proportion to each other, so varies the softness of the end- product for its intended application, because maxillofacial prosthetics tend to require greater softness and flexibility.

Epithane-3 and Calthane are the only polyurethanes currently available for fabricating facial prostheses.

These are three component, room-temperature curing system .

These can be used to restore defects with mobile tissue beds as the positive qualities of this material pertain to its flexibility without losing strength at the edges, which allows margins to be made thin to obtain optimal esthetics.

These have inherent environmental Silicone and methyl chloride react to form dimethyldichlorosilane.

When water is added to dimethyldichlorosilane, a fluid polymer, polydimethyl siloxane (PDMS), is formed that is white and translucent and of varying viscosity, which is determined by the length of the polymer .

The PDMS chains and the silica fillers and the interactions between these two components affect the overall strength and service life of the silicone based maxillofacial prosthetic material.

To increase the strength various types of fillers are added to reinforce the elastomers. Fumed silica, precipitated silica, aero gels are the most frequently used silica with the silicones. Polysiloxanes must be cross-linked to form solid elastomer materials. Antioxidants and vulcanizing agents are added to change the raw mass into rubbery resins during processing and the process of cross linking is known as vulcanizing.

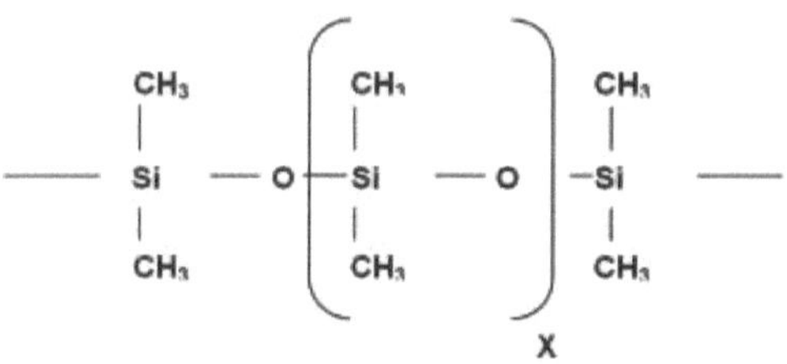

Where X is the degree of polymerization

Polydimethyl Siloxane

HTV silicone Heat:

-vulcanized silicones are used occasionally for maxillofacial prostheses.

It is usually a white, opaque material with a highly viscous, and putty like consistency.

It is available as one component or two component putty.

The vulcanization mechanism is achieved by an addition reaction.

The components of heat-vulcanized silicones are a polydimethylvinyl siloxane copolymer with approximately 0.5% vinyl side chains, 2,4- dichlorobenzoyl peroxide as an initiator(vulcanizing agent) ,and a silica filler obtained from burning methyl silane.

Catalyst of HTV is platinum salt (salt of chloroplatinic acid)linking, however requires water molecules to hydrolyze the silane and produces acetic acid (an irritant) as the by-product. The use has therefore been limited to that of an extrinsic colourant carrier applied to the surface of the prosthesis. [36]

Advantages:-

- Excellent tear strength and highest tensile
- Strength at 5.87 MPa (polyurethane the lowest at 0.83 MPa.).
- Excellent thermal
- Colour
- Chemical stability (rendering it more biologically inert)
- High percent elongation.

Disadvantages:

- Poor esthetics due to opacity.
- Less elasticity.
- Low edge strength.
- Technique sensitive. [37]

Stephen M. Parel, Per-Ingvar Brånemark, MD, PhD, Lars-Olof Ohrnell, and Barbro Svensson narrated that The rehabilitation of maxillary defects is a significant challenge in terms of creating retention and preserving existing dentition in an environment of expanded functional stress. The advent of osseointegration has enhanced the dental practitioner's capabilities in this regard with a remarkably improved potential for increasing prosthesis stability and preserving tissue. For patients with extensive prosthetic cantilevers, however, the opportunity for implant placement in defect areas is compromised unless remote bone sites are considered. Implants in the defect buttress zone through the maxillary sinus in non-defect sites (zygoma implants) can be valuable in providing a level of functional rehabilitation previously unattainable.[7]

Faysal Ugurlu, Coskun YJldJz, B. C. Sener, and Atilla Sertgoz narrated that Zygomatic implants have been used for dental rehabilitation in patients with insufficient bone in the posterior upper jaw, due to, for example, tumor resection, trauma, or atrophy. Zygomatic implants are an alternative to complex free or vascularized bone grafting and distraction osteogenesis. A 42-year-old male patient with a severe defect in the right posterior maxilla, starting from the first canine region, which had occurred after tumor resection 3 years earlier, was referred to our department. One zygomatic implant (Brenemark System, Nobel Biocare, Goteborg, Sweden) to the zygoma and one dental implant to the canine region were placed. After a 5-month osseointegration period, a fixed denture was fabricated and adapted to the implants. Although the surgical and prosthetic procedures for zygoma implants are not easy, the final outcomes can be successful with appropriate planning.[10]

The study was conducted by G. Pekkan, S.H. Tuna, F. Oghan in 2011 to evaluate extraoral prostheses and the use of extraoral implants in patients with facial defects. 10 cases were treated utilizing maxillofacial prostheses employing extraoral implants in five cases. 16 extraoral implants were installed. Seven implants were placed in irradiated sites in the orbital regions. Six implants were placed in mastoid regions and three in a zygoma region that was irradiated. Two implants failed before initial integration was achieved in irradiated areas. Using 14 extraoral implants as anchors, five extraoral prostheses were set. The other five cases were treated with extraoral prostheses without using extraoral implants due to cost and patient-related factors. The data included age, sex, primary disease, implant length, implant failure, prosthetic attachment, radiation therapy, and peri-implant skin reactions. The study concluded that the use of extraoral implants for the retention of extraoral prostheses has simplified the placement, removal, and cleaning of the prosthesis by the patient. The stability of the prostheses was improved by anchors. Clinical and technical problems are presented with the techniques used for their resolution. Using extraoral implants resulted in a high rate of success in retaining facial prostheses and gave good stability and aesthetic satisfaction.[12]

Sumayya A Nazar, Dr. Vivek V Nair, Dr. Harsha Kumar K and Dr. R Ravichandran in their review article narrated that the facial region defects caused by trauma, accident, tumour or congenital defects are treated with maxillofacial prostheses. A part from esthetics, the most common problem encountered with these prostheses is the retention of prostheses. The success of maxillofacial prostheses in meeting the expectations of patients and prosthodontists is on rise with the development of adhesive material science, the emergence of technical knowledge, and the development of implant technology. Increase in retention provides ease of use and psychological acceptance by the patient thereby improving the long-term prognosis of the prosthesis. In this review, the methods used for the retention of prostheses from past to present along with the advantages of adhesives and implants, implementation of 3D technology and rapid prototyping were critically appraised.[15]

The clinical report was conducted by David Faustino Ângelo,José Ricardo Vieira Ferreira in which the 44-year-old male patient had history of congenital dental agenesis. A previous oral rehabilitation with an all-on-6 type, implant-fixed

mandibular overdenture, had failed due to peri-implantitis. The patient was successfully treated with bimaxillary custom made subperiosteal implants with an innovative design, combining subperiosteal and endosseous support.
The authors consider custom-made subperiosteal implants, in selected patients, present several advantages over classic bone-grafting plus endosseous implant-placement techniques such as (1) possibility of a single-stage procedure with immediate loading in atrophic jaws; (2) possible primary option to approach atrophic jaws as a simpler and less time-consuming technique; and (3) a valid rescue option for failed endosseous implants.[16]

A case report was obtained by Borgia Gonzalo , Ravecca Tabaré, Fumero Miriam , Pebé Pablo from the department of Oral and Maxillofacial Implantology to observe the use of osseointegrated implants as an effective and safe anchorage tool for oral-maxillofacial prostheses. The conclusion derived was the design of tapered dental implants, with a reduced platform, is suitable for this low density and limited width region.[19]

The study was conducted by Aleix Solà Pérez , David Pastorino , Carlos Aparicio , Marta Pegueroles Neyra , Rabia Sannam Khan, Simon Wright and Cemal Ucer A systematic review of the literature on zygomatic implant for the treatment of severe maxillary atrophy was performed and 196 publications were included in the study. The cumulative success rate of zygomatic implants for the treatment of severe maxillary atrophy was 98.5% at less than 1 year, 97.5% between 1 and 3 years, 96.8% between 3 and 5 years and 96.1% after more than 5 years. The most commonly reported complications were soft tissue dehiscence, rhinosinusitis and prosthetic failures. The treatment of severe lack of bone in the upper maxilla with zygomatic implants is a safe procedure, reaching a cumulative success rate of 96.1% after more than 5 years.[20]

A Clinical case done was done by Marion E. Kreissl, DDS, Dr meddent, Guido Heydecke, Marc C. Metzger, and Ralf Schoen, habil School of Dentistry, University Hospital, Freiburg, Germany. In the clinical report, a diabetic patient with a status of posthemimaxillectomy secondary to aspergillusis infection is presented, in whom a zygoma implant was placed using a CT scan–based navigation system. A special retentive anchoring abutment was used to integrate the zygoma implant into a telescopic crown–retained denture on the residual dentition. This tooth-implant-supported obturator prosthesis restored function and phonetics, as well as esthetics, for this young patient.[21]

The clinical case study conducted by Elizabeth Alfenas , Isadora Silva, Davidson Oliveira , Paul Tanner, Francisca Jardilino describes the unique and highly-specialized fabrication method of an oral and facial prosthesis for a patient with a near total maxillectomy, excision of upper lip, rhinectomy and radiotherapy for treatment of an extensive malignant neoplasm. Four carefully placed zygomatic implants were used to retain an oral obturator and an external mid-facial prosthesis. The prosthetic rehabilitation allowed the patient's reintegration into society accompanying the satisfactory restoration of aesthetics, phonetics, mastication, and deglutition.[23]

V Jain , Modhupa Ghosh , Ruchi Goel , Rekha Gupta , Priyanka Golhait , Basudeb Ghosh conducted a clinical report highlighting the challenges faced in planning, designing and placement of maxillofacial implants in the supra-orbital rim of an exenterated socket post-radiotherapy along with the management of the unexpected complications which developed subsequently. Administration of hyperbaric oxygen therapy, fabrication of a digitally designed surgical guide to ensure predictable implant placement, selection of surface treated implants for better biomechanical anchorage, and a gentler surgical technique for recovery of irradiated hard and soft tissues were measures undertaken during the treatment phase. An effort has been made to point-out the fact that despite the various approaches adopted in an irradiated patient, success of implant placement in such a situation remains a challenge.[26]

The study was conducted by Guido R. Sigron , Nathalie Rüedi , Frédérique Chammartin , Simon Meyer , Bilal Msallem , et al to compare the efficacy of the intraoperative bending of titanium mesh with the efficacy of pre-contoured "hybrid" patient-specific titanium mesh for the surgical repair of isolated orbital floor fractures. The first twelve patients underwent conventional reconstruction with intraoperative free-hand bending of an orbital floor mesh plate. The subsequent ten patients received pre-contoured plates based on 3D-printed orbital models that were produced by mirroring the non-fractured orbit of the patient using a medical imaging software. The study concluded that the use of 3D-printed orbital models leads to a more accurate reconstruction and a time reduction during surgery.[27]

A study was conducted by N. Fontaine , P. Hemar , P. Schultz , A. Charpiot , C. Debry in 2013 . The objective of this study was to compare two operative techniques: skin flap, and full-thickness skin graft. Material and methods: Between January 2004 and January 2011, 72 patients were treated by BAHA implant and 32 of these patients (total of 41 implants) were included in the study. Two surgical techniques were used: full-thickness skin graft (n = 21) and skin flap (n = 20) Results: Four types of skin complications were observed: necrosis, inflammation/infection, hypertrophic scar, and fixture loss due to inadequate osseointegration. Complications requiring surgical revision were observed in 20% of cases with the skin flap method and 38% of cases with the skin graft technique, with no significant difference between the two groups. The study concluded that : The skin graft technique appeared to be associated with a higher rate of major complications. The most common complication is hypertrophic scar.[34]

The study was conducted by Naseer Alsseri and Ahmed Alasraj stated : Reconstructing maxillofacial defects is quite challenging for most surgeons due to the region's complex anatomy and cosmetic and functional effects on patients. The use of pre-made alloplastic implants and autogenous grafts is often associated with resorption, infection, and displacement. Recent technological advances have led to the use of custom computer-designed patient-specific implants (PSIs) in reconstructive surgery.[35]

The study was done by Krishna Patel, Kathleyn Brandstetter ,stating the effective use of implants to reconstruct a variety of bony and soft-tissue defects, including the frontal and temporal regions; internal orbit; infraorbital rim; malar, paranasal, and nasal regions; mandible; and chin. The study concluded that ,In comparison to their autologous counterparts, alloplastic materials are more readily available, lack donor site morbidity, decrease surgical time and cost, and still have relatively good postoperative tissue tolerance.[38]

A Study was conducted by Kiran Patel, Sonal Madan, Deval Mehta, Setu P. Shah, Vaibhav Trivedi, Hemant Seta in 2021 . The aim of the study was to conduct a prospective evaluation for the feasibility of placing strategic basal implants in clinical practice along with its merits and demerits. s. Materials and Methods: A prospective study was designed to evaluate the protocol of immediate functional loading using the technology of strategic basal implants for fixed complete arch prostheses and segmental teeth prostheses. Aminimal of 10 patients selected in the age group of 20–80 years were restored with strategic basal implants irrespective of the quality and quantity of cancellous/alveolar bone following immediate functional loading protocols. Results: About 157 various designs of basal implants were placed in 10 patients, out of which four failed with the survival rate of 97.5% of basal implants.[41]

The study was conducted by AA Diken Türksayar, SA Saglam, AC Bulut in the year 2019, the methods used for the retention of prostheses from past to present were researched, and the advantages of adhesives and implants, which are the most commonly used current methods, were evaluated. The study concluded that according to the area where the facial prosthesis will be applied, the presence of different implant systems with bar holders or magnetic holders provides maximum retention and comfort of use.[43]

A study was conducted by L. Vrielinck, C. Politis, S. Schepers, M. Pauwels, I. Naert in 2003. The aim of the study was to present and validate a planning system for implant insertion based on preoperative CT imaging. It allowed the surgeon to determine the desired position of different kinds of implants. Finally a customized drill guide was produced by stereolithography. In this study, zygoma, pterygoid and regular platform implants were used. The treatment protocol was validated through 12 case studies, selected at random from the total patient group (n=29 patients). From postoperative images, the exact implant location was determined and the deviation of axes between planned and inserted implants was calculated. In this in vivo study, displacements, varying according to the type of implant and the location of the implants, were observed. From a clinical standpoint, most of the inserted implants were judged to be adequately sited. A prospective clinical follow-up study was performed on all 29 patients. The study concluded that eventhough all patients presented with severe maxillary atrophy, excellent cumulative survival rates (92%) for the zygoma implants and 93% for regular platform implants was obtained.[45]

A clinical study was conducted by Faysal Ugurlu, Coskun YJldJz, B. C. Sener, and Atilla Sertgoz of 42-year-old male patient with a severe defect in the right posterior maxilla, starting from the first canine region, which had occurred after tumor resection 3 years earlier. One zygomatic implant (Brenemark System, Nobel Biocare, Goteborg, Sweden) to the zygoma and one dental implant to the canine region were placed. After a 5-month osseointegration period, a fixed denture was fabricated and adapted to the implants. The study concluded that ,although the surgical and prosthetic procedures for zygoma implants were not easy, the final outcomes were successful with appropriate planning.[46]

A study was conducted by Sailesh Kumar Mukul, Madan Mishra, Gaurav Singh, Abhishek Singh and Manthan Kumar Das to evaluate the need to reconstruct the defect in the most precise way for the surgical procedure for enhancing patient outcomes and well-being. The introduction of 3-dimensional printing in the biomedical field had led to the utilization of patient-specific implants (PSIs) in the surgical repair of maxillofacial defects, which occur congenitally, posttraumatically, or postsurgically. PSI fit quickly with greater accuracy with the added benefit of shorter rehabilitation time. Material and Method: A 21-year-old male with a history of left zygomatico–orbital–maxillary complex fracture presented complaining of secondary deformity as a result of facial trauma. He underwent zygomatic osteotomy and repositioning followed by PSI reconstruction of the left zygoma, left orbital floor with titanium implants. A hemicoronal, subcilliary, and maxillary vestibular approaches were used. Result: Good esthetic results with no postoperative complications are obtained. The study concluded that the use of PSI for the reconstruction of oral and craniomaxillofacial defects should be considered an accurate alternative to noncustom-made implants. Automation allows for the application of safe, time-effective procedures not requiring specialized, and software-specific knowledge.[47]

RECENT ADVANCES IN MAXILLOFACIAL PROSTHESES

The use of Computed Tomography (CT) and Magnetic Resonance Imaging (MRI) in conjunction with Rapid Prototyping (RP) have revolutionized the methods of old-fashioned impressions using various types of dental materials and sculpting of the prosthesis by hand in wax or clay .[32]

Recently advances in 3D optical imaging using 3D whole field profilometer based on the projection of incoherent light and 3D laser eye-safe scanners have been utilized . The advantages of such a system are that they are non-invasive, have a higher speed of data acquisition, and the scanners are more rugged and portable than the CT or MRI scanners.

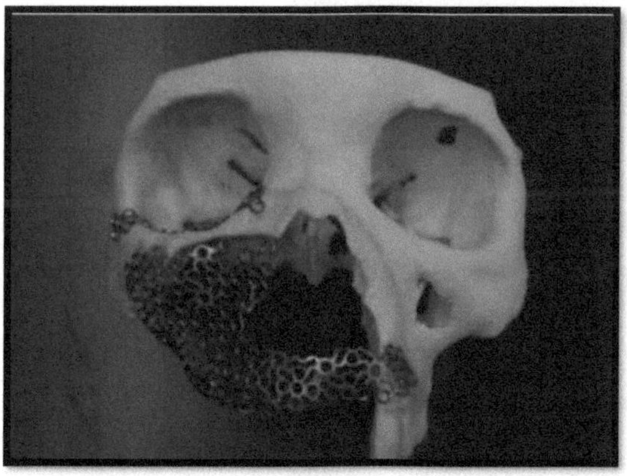

FIGURE:70

Rapid prototype modelling of maxillofacial prosthesis

Once the data has been acquired the virtual 3D models are obtained and the final prosthesis can be designed virtually.

Two models one with the defect and another with the built up prosthesis are generated using epoxy photo-polymerising resins in a 3D printer .The final prosthesis is then fabricated from silicone rubber using these moulds.

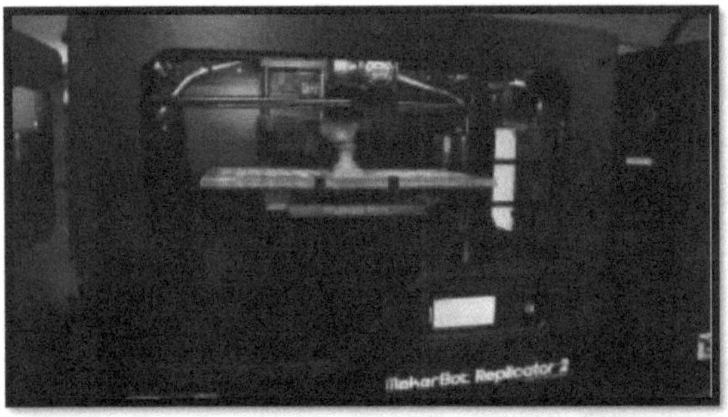

3D PRINTER

FIGURE:71

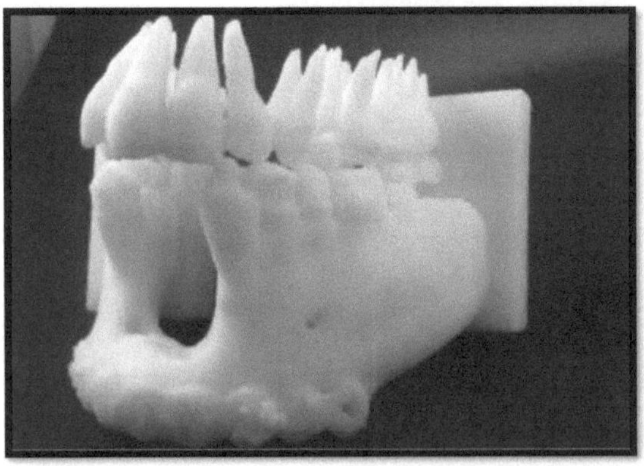

3D printer model of mandibular defect

FIGURE:72

In order to minimize the harmful effects of the metallic implants and their by-products, several newer materials are being tried.

New alloys like **tantalum, niobium, zirconium, and magnesium** are receiving attention given their satisfying mechanical and biological properties.

Non-oxide ceramics like silicon nitride and silicon carbide are being currently developed as a promising implant material possessing a combination of properties such as good wear and corrosion resistance, increased ductility, good fracture and creep resistance, and relatively high hardness in comparison to alumina.

Polymer/magnesium composites are being developed to improve mechanical properties as well as retain polymer's property of degradation .

Nanotechnology and tissue engineering along with the concepts of stem cell technology are poised to dramatically define the next quantum leap in the field of maxillofacial reconstruction.

Whether it is regeneration of new osseous tissue in vivo for placement of implants or even the regeneration of a complete ear or nose literally 'grown' from the stem cells of the person or a suitable donor-the possibilities are endless .

It seems to be just a matter of time before the dream of autologous reconstruction of defective or missing anatomical structures soon becomes a reality.[40]

Extraoral implants in mastoid region have very high success rate near to 100%. The implant-retained facial prosthesis provides more satisfaction rather than adhesive retained due to ease of use and proper retention in daily activities.[6]

Implants commonly used in facial prosthesis are extraoral implants which are much more expensive than conventional dental implants. Patients with maxillofacial defects often have financial burdens because these patients often are unemployed as a result of their diseases. The dental implant was used because of financial considerations and better accessibility of dental implant components in surgery and prosthesis procedures. Patient had properly large deficiency so longer 6 mm dental implants had some advantages versus short 3 mm extra oral implants to provide proper anchorage for this heavy auricular prosthesis. Use of bar and bridge abutment in the role of transcutaneous component was done and because of fixation with an independent screw, other steps could be run without need to take out of this transcutaneous component. Placement of implants in antihelix part of future auricular prosthesis caused hiding of retentive components easy and provided esthetic and natural view which was accessed through a surgical stent which mimics final auricular prosthesis. The advantages of extraoral implants are numerous, they provide consistent retention and positioning of the facial prosthesis and can be placed during the primary reconstruction procedure or anytime postoperatively when the patient can tolerate the procedure.

In addition to providing predictable retention, several other important advantages were achieved . [8]

The aesthetics and durability of prostheses have been enhanced because fine feathered margins are maintainable and not liable to damage by adhesives and solvent.

Patients with oral malignancies are often treated with surgery followed by radiation therapy.

Once irradiated, the bone's potential for implant placement can be compromised severely or lost because its osteogenic potential and microvascularity are decreased.

Adjunctive therapies such as hyperbaric oxygen treatment and subsequent implant placement in irradiated bone have been proposed.

The influence of hyperbaric oxygen therapy remains uncertain but promising .

The effects of irradiation on the cellular and structural components of bone and the overlying soft tissues are well known but the possible effects of irradiation on the prognosis of endosseous implant therapy and on the process of osseointegration are controversial.

The success rates in irradiated patients are far lower and vary with anatomical location.

Their study indicated that the success rate of orbital implants in patients who had not received radiotherapy was 94%.

The implant success rate in irradiated patients was 61%. The success rates in the midface and in radiated patients proved more variable.

WOLFAARDT et al. reported a 69% success rate for extra-oral implants inserted in irradiated patients.

Intraoral implants are connected through the oral mucosa, which is bathed in saliva, providing a tenacious protective environment for the soft tissue–abutment interface. In the case of extraoral implants, the biological and mechanical milieu is very different.

The osseous encasement of the extraoral implant varies greatly between regions, and the length of the implants is far shorter than that of intraoral implants. [11]

The loads applied to extraoral implants are different and the connection through the skin to the external environment provides a totally different soft tissue environment for the abutment. [9]

Extraoral implants can only be evaluated by assessing implant immobility and the peri-abutment skin reaction; they cannot be routinely radiographed.

The skin around the implants must be cared for regularly by the patients, with daily cleansing combined with adjustments by the clinician at follow-up visits.

Once implants are successfully placed, three basic retentive systems can be used: the bar and clip, the ball and keeper, and the magnet and keeper.

The bars and clips, can be utilized for each patient to ensure mechanical advantage. Disadvantages are the cost and the increased difficulty for the patient in performing the necessary implant-associated hygiene. GRANSTRO¨ M et al. pointed out that the use of bars and clips attached to implants to facilitate positioning of the prosthesis limits ease of use, implant hygiene and there is a risk of fracture with a significantly negative effect on implant survival.[12]

The ball and keeper and magnet and keeper systems are easy to use. They require no special laboratory procedures, which reduces costs. They can be cleaned easily by the patient and maintained by the dentist.

The use of magnets is advantageous compared with conventional bars and clips, because magnetic retention creates relatively low moment forces on the supporting abutment, allowing easy hygiene control and removal of the prosthesis by the patient

.

In most instances, they are placed in a straight line, which may decrease stability.

The incidence of facial sites treated with implant-supported prostheses indicated that the auricular (72%) region was the most common site, followed by the orbital (20%), nasal (6%), and combination (2%).

Clips were the predominant mechanism used to retain auricular prostheses.[29]

Orbital prostheses were fabricated with a wider variety and combination of attachments. The results of this survey indicate a need for further investigation regarding the most efficacious attachment method for patients treated with implant-supported facial prostheses.

In this study, patient satisfaction was higher with implant-retained prostheses than with conventional adhesive retained ones. [11]

In patients without implants, prosthetic retention was achieved using tissue undercuts such as orbital socket and external auditory canal, eye glasses, and skin adhesives.

Implant patients benefited from bars and magnetic attachments. Adhesive-retained facial prostheses had to be remade more frequently than the implant-retained ones due to the discolouration and deterioration of the silicone prosthesis after frequent use of the adhesives and solvents.

The prosthetic challenges were mainly the fabrication of the ocular prostheses and attachment between the silicone prosthesis and the acrylic template (acrylic resin substructure), which was made to attach the sleeve of the bar or magnet keeper.[14]

An **orbital prosthesis** helps camouflage lost structures and provides a semblance of esthetic, morphological, functional and psychological normality in those affected.[24]

The conventional means of anchorage for maxillofacial prosthesis encompass anatomical undercuts, tissue adhesives, double sided tapes, spectacle frames, and magnets.

However, the composite nature of the defect, its large size, and the absence of suitable anatomical undercuts in the patient mandated an additional retentive source for a definitive orbital prosthesis. Surgical anchorage by means of osseointegrated craniofacial implants provides a significant advantage in terms of prosthesis retention, stability, placement, and longevity along with improved accessibility for optimal tumor aftercare.[39]

MATERIALS IN MAXILLOFACIAL PROSTHESES

Maxillofacial defects are difficult to treat due to their important functional, esthetic, and psychological aspects.

The anatomical complexity of this region has also contributed to the challenge it presents all surgeons, including veterans.

Traditional pre-made implants often require many adjustments and usually offer suboptimal results .

The advances made in AM technology as well as 3D imaging have contributed greatly to the management of maxillofacial defects. This has facilitated the manufacturing of custom-made PSI that mirrors the healthy side to achieve a satisfactory result.

Computer-designed PSI offers higher accuracy and defect adaption, enhanced stability, more predictable outcomes, and better facial contour refinement . Premade alloplastic implants usually require major intraoperative adjustments for large complex defects. In the literature, the usual complications associated with other materials, such as infection, foreign body reaction, and displacement, are seldom reported in relation to custommade PSI . [36]

Using AM technology, it was able to operate on 6 patients with various maxillofacial defects using a total of 8 PEEKs and 2 titanium PSIs. Initially ,challenges were faced meeting the requirements for completing proper preoperative CT for 3D planning. This was solved by always requesting 1–mm-thick CT for all PSI cases.

When designing custom-made PSI, engineers tend to design fixation screw holes in the area where the thickest bone is found irrespective of any vital tissues in the area.

However, **it is easy to drill wherever it is more preferable in the final implant regardless of the pre-designed screw hole**.

This is one of the advantages of using PEEK versus pre-made alloplastic implants such as **silicone.** [31]

It is not possible to drill a screw hole anywhere other than the pre-designed screw hole; doing so otherwise would lead to implant tearing and loss. One of the challenges faced was fixing mandibular angle PSI. [37]

In preformed alloplastic implants, the superior border is usually extended near the dentition to facilitate the fixation process. However, since PSI is based on mirroring of the healthy side, the superior portion is usually located near the inferior border of the mandible or middle part of the lateral cortex. We believe that this issue could be solved by planning all mandibular angle PSIs to have an extended superior border with a minimum thickness to facilitate the fixation process. PEEK was used to fabricate 8 of the 10 PSIs used here. The use of PEEK in reconstructive surgery is well documented in the literature owing to its excellent biocompatibility, adjustability, stability, chemical inertness, radiolucency, and mechanical properties. In reconstructing the secondary deformity involving the zygoma and orbit, custom-made titanium implant was used in the orbit instead of PEEK because it is more affordable, and no further adjustments would be needed.

The zygoma was reconstructed using a separate PEEK PSI. According to the experience shared , the PSI we used required minimal adjustments that were easily made intraoperatively.

However, it should be noted that many issues were faced inserting larger implants, requiring the extension of our surgical approach. It was concluded that this could be easily alleviated by separating larger implants into separate smaller pieces with connectors in between .

A major issue faced was designing custom implants for the **nasal area**. This problem stemmed from the fact that it was impossible to mirror the healthy side since the entire bone was affected.[29]

To overcome this limitation, an average of healthy nasal bones was taken and implemented into the final design. However, the resulting implant was too bulky and required further intraoperative adjustments.

Hence, The use of PSI for maxillofacial reconstruction features predictable outcomes, eliminates the usual complications seen in non-custom-made implants, and boasts excellent patient satisfaction with high cost as the main drawback.[37]

Maxillofacial prostheses play a vital role in comprehensive rehabilitation by restoring physical and psychological well-being in patients with missing or disfigured anatomical structures due to congenital abnormalities, trauma or disease.

It is possible to restore esthetics, function and re establish the self confidence of the patient by providing a well designed prosthesis such as a prosthetic ear, eye, nose, cranial plate or a combination of these.

It is necessary to have a clear concept about the science of implantation and the healing of bone following a successsful implant placement. Various surface modifications like grit blasting and acid etching are widely used.

Craniofacial implants require adequate osseous thickness of the bone on the temporal and mastoid regions . Implant placement may not be as ideal in normal situations or with acquired defects from accidents.

Other crucial factors in rehabilitation are marginal fit, good retention, and acceptable esthetics.

In future it is hoped that technological advances in allied field such as radioodiagnosis and imaging, CAD-CAM manufacturing ,tissue engineering, laser scanning, will work in tandem to ensure that enlarger numbers of patients can be treated early, economically and effectively.

The discovery of osseointegration has been arguably one of the most beneficial medical breakthroughs especially in the head and neck region.
The number of successful implants being placed is increasing rapidly as better implants, more efficient investigative techniques and superior armamentarium is readily available.
These implants have also revolutionized the scope and the efficacy of rehabilitation of the entire craniofacial region.
Despite the rise in cancers of the head and neck region there is also a deeper understanding of the changes at cellular level and better treatment options and targeted medication.
It is hoped that with each passing day there will be continued dedicated research to fight and eradicate all these killer diseases. Until then the science of craniofacial implantology will ensure that the patients receive the most comprehensive rehabilitation that can be offered and ensure that their early return to form and function.
In future it is hoped that technological advances in allied fields such as radio-diagnosis and imaging, CAD-CAM manufacturing, tissue engineering, laser scanning, 3D-printing, development of newer nano-based materials and robotic placement of implants will work in tandem to ensure that larger numbers of patients can be treated early, economically and effectively .
Then alone will the dream of health for all be truly a reality.

1. The Glossary of Prosthodontic Terms 2023: Tenth Edition. J Prosthet Dent. 2023 Oct;130.
2. Chalian VA, Drane JB, Standish SM. Maxillofacial Prosthetics. Baltimore: The Williams and Wilkins Co.; 1971.
3. Fernanda Pereira de Caxias, Daniela Micheline , Lisiane Bannwart. Classification, History and Future Prospects of Maxillofacial Prosthesis. Int J Dent. 2019;Jul:18.
4. Durrani Z, Hussain SG, Alam S A. A Study of Classification Systems for Maxillectomy Defects. JPPA 2013; 01(02): 117-124.
5. Hovhannisyan s. R., mashinyan k. A., zopunyan v. R. Maxillofacial defects
6. Cawood, J.I.; Howell, R.A. Reconstructive preprosthetic surgery. I. Anatomical considerations. Int. J. Oral Maxillofac. Surg. 1991,20;75–82.
7. Branemark PI. Osseointegration and its experimental background. J Prosthet Dent. 1983;50:399-410.
8. Role of Implants in maxillofacial prosthodontic rehabilitation by Derek D' Souza.
9. Jacobsson M, Tjellstrom A, Fine L, et al: A retrospective study of osseointegrated skin-penetrating titanium fixtures used for retaining facial prostheses. Int J Oral Maxillofac Implants 1992;07:523.
10. Chang TL, Garrett N, Roumanas E, et al. Treatment satisfaction with facial prostheses. J Prosthet Dent. 2005;94:275-80.
11. Leonardi A, Buonaccorsi S, Pellacchia V, et al: Maxillofacial prosthetic rehabilitation using extraoral implants. J Craniofac Surg.2008;19:398.
12. G. Pekkan, S.H. Tuna, F. Oghan: Extraoral prostheses using extraoral implants. Int. J. Oral Maxillofac. Surg. 2011; 40: 378–383
13. Anita Visser, M. Raghoebar, Robert P. Van Oort, ArjanVissink; Fate of Implant Retained Craniofacial Prosthesis: Life Span and Aftercare; The International Journal Oral and Maxillofacial Implants.2008; 23:1.
14. C. Sabarigirinathan, Implants in Maxillofacial Prosthesis ; Journal of Science ,2015; 5(12): 1131-1136.
15. Ghalaut P, Shekhawat H ,Meena B. Full-mouth rehabilitation with immediate loading basal implants: A case report. Natl J Maxillofac Surg. 2019 Jan-Jun;10(1):91.

16. Angelo DF, Vieira Ferreira JR. The Role of Custom-made Subperiosteal Implants for Rehabilitation of Atrophic Jaws- Case Report. Ann Maxillofac Surg. 2020;10(2):507-511.
17. Subperiosteal Dental Implants-Instituto Maxillofacial Orthognathic Surgery and Implantology.
18. Atalay, B.; Do ˘ganay, Ö.; Saraço ˘glu, B.K.; Bultan, Ö.; Hafiz, G. Clinical Evaluation of Zygomatic Implant-Supported Fixed and Removable Prosthesis. J. Craniofacial Surg. 2017, 28, 185–189
19. Aparicio C, Manresa C, Francisco K, Ouazzani W, Claros P, Potau JM, et al. The long-term use of zygomatic implants: A 10-year clinical and radiographic report. Clin Implant Dent Relat Res 2014;16:447-59.
20. Davo R, Malevez C, Pons O. Immediately loaded zygomatic implants: a 5-year prospective study.J Oral Implantology.2013;(6):39.
21. Meenakshi, DS. The obturator prostheses for maxillectomy A SRM J Res. Dent Sci 2012;3:193-7.
22. Takafumi Otomaru, Yuka I, Sumita. Rehabilitation of a bilateral maxillectomy patient with a free fibula osteocutaneous flap and with an implant-retained obturator: a clinical report. J Prosthet Dent. 2015. Jan;11.
23. Gowda ME , Mohan MS, Verma K ,Roy ID .Implant rehabilitation of partial maxillectomy edentulous patient. Contemp Clin Dent. 2013;4(3):39.
24. Sompop Bencharit, Challenges and Prospective Applications of Extra-oral Implants for Maxillofacial Rehabilitation; Anaplastology 2012;1(2).
25. Toljanic JA, Eckert SE, Roumanas E, et al. Osseointegrated craniofacial implants in the rehabilitation of orbital defects: an update of a retrospective experience in the United States. J Prosthet Dent. 2005;94:177–182.
26. Pruthi G, Jain V, Sikka S. A novel method for retention of an orbital prosthesis in a case with continuous maxillary and orbital defect. J Indian Prosthodont Soc. 2010;10: 132–136.
27. Sigron GR, Ruedi N, Chammartin F, Meyer S , Kunz C ,Thieringer FM. Three-Dimensional Analysis of Isolated Orbital Floor Fractures Pre- and Post-

Reconstruction with Standard Titanium Meshes and "Hybrid" Patient-Specific Implants, J Clin Med. 2020 May.

28. Jensen OT, Brownd C, Blacker J: Nasofacial prostheses supported by osseointegrated implants. Int J Oral Maxillofac Implants.1992;7:203.
29. Balaghi F, Hasanzade M, Zarati S. Implant-retained Nasal Prosthesis with Bar and Clip for a Patient with Total Rhinectomy: A Clinical Report. Front Dent .2019;16(6):47.
30. Cemal Aydin; Implant – Retained Auricular Prosthesis: An Assessment of Implant Success and Prosthestic Complications; The International Journal of Prosthodontics.2008;21:3.
31. Lemon JC, Chambers MS. Locking retentive attachment for an implant-retained auricular prosthesis. N Y State Dent J. 1999;65:26-31.
32. VJ, Stephens WF. Prosthetic rehabilitation of an extensive midfacial and palatal postsurgical defect with an implant-supported cross arch framework: A clinical report. J Prosthet Dent. 2015;113:502.
33. Hagr A. BAHA : Bone-Anchored Hearing Aid .Int J Health Sci(Qassim). 2007;1(2):26.
34. Bento RF ,Kiesewetter A , Ikari LS ,Brito R. Bone-anchored hearing aid (BAHA): indications, functional results , and comparison with reconstructive surgery of the ear. Int Arch Otorhinolaryngol. 2012;16(3):40.
35. Kim MM, Boahene KD, Byrne PJ (2009) Use of customized polyetheretherketone (PEEK) implants in the reconstruction of complex maxillofacial defects. Arch Facial Plast Surg 11(1):53–57.
36. Scolozzi P, Martinez A, Jaques B (2007) Complex orbito-fronto-temporal reconstruction using computer-designed PEEK implant. J Craniofac Surg 18(1):224–228.
37. Wong JK Forehead augmentation with alloplastic implants. Facial Plast Surg Clin North Am.2010;18(1):71.
38. Patel K, Brandstetter K. Solid implants in Facial Plastic Surgery: Potential Complications and How to Prevent Them. Facial Plast Surg. 2016;32(5):52.

39. Terino EO, Edwards MC .Customizing jawlines :the art of alloplastic premandible contouring . Facial Plast Surg Clin North Am. 2008;16(1):99.
40. Corina ,Loana T, Alessandro L. Digital workflow in maxillofacial prosthodontics – An Update on Defect Data Acquisition, Editing and Design Using Open source Software.2021.18;(4)97.
41. Patel K, Madan S, Mehta D, Shah SP, Trivedi V, Seta H. Basal implants: An asset for rehabilitation of atrophied resorbed maxillary and mandibular jaw – A prospective study. Ann Maxillofac Surg 2021;11:64-9.
42. Solà Pérez, A.; Pastorino, D.; Aparicio, C.; Pegueroles Neyra, M.; Khan, R.S.; Wright, S.; Ucer, C. Success Rates of Zygomatic Implants for the Rehabilitation of Severely Atrophic Maxilla: A Systematic Review. Dent. J. 2022;10:151.
43. Diken Türksayar AA, Saglam SA, Bulut AC. Retention systems used in maxillofacial prostheses: A review. Niger J Clin Pract 2019;22:16.
44. Tessier P. The definitive plastic surgical treatment of the severe facial deformities of craniofacial dysostosis: Crouzon and Apert's diseases. Plast Reconstr Surg 1971;48:41.
45. L. Vrielinck, C. Politis, S. Schepers, M. Pauwels, I. Naert: Image-based planning and clinical validation of zygoma and pterygoid implant placement in patients with severe bone atrophy using customized drill guides. Preliminary results from a prospective clinical follow-up study. Int. J. Oral Maxillofac. Surg. 2003; 32: 7–14.
46. Faysal Ugurlu, Coskun YJldJz, B. C. Sener, and Atilla Sertgo .Rehabilitation of Posterior Maxilla with Zygomatic and Dental Implant after Tumor Resection: A Case Report Hindawi Publishing Corporation;2013;3.
47. Sailesh Kumar Mukul1, Madan Mishra2, Gaurav Singh2, Abhishek Singh2 and Manthan Kumar Das Patient-Specific Implants in Maxillofacial Reconstruction: A Case Report .sage journal 2022;1.

FSC
www.fsc.org
MIX
Papier | Fördert gute Waldnutzung
FSC® C083411

Kolibri 360 GmbH
Ferdinand-Jühlke-Straße 7
99095 Erfurt, Deutschland
produktsicherheit@kolibri360.de

Druck:
CPI Druckdienstleistungen GmbH
im Auftrag der
Kolibri 360 GmbH
Ferdinand-Jühlke-Str. 7
99095 Erfurt